5 Star review

✓ I am so very glad I bought this book as it has definitely given me a great insight into dementia and has hopefully helped me understand the potential issues involved when looking after my elderly relatives. Hopefully, I will be more patient and compassionate in the future. The real-life journey interspersed with helpful facts has desensitised a difficult and shunned subject, and I will definitely be recommending this to everyone I know who has connections with any type of dementia.

✓ My husband has Parkinson's and what I believe to be DLB. Thank you for sharing your experiences about this awful disease. I saw a reference to your book and downloaded it, which was probably the best thing I've done for a long time. I will now be able to deal with things in a much more sensitive way. Thank you so much. I would recommend this book to everyone who has to deal with DLB. It is an invaluable source of help and comfort.

✓ This book has already been invaluable to me. My dad was diagnosed this week with LBD. This book has helped me make sense of his symptoms, given me good information about the disease, the other types of dementia and the difference and given me some hope for the road ahead. But it's also not sugar-coated what to possibly expect, how to have some coping strategies, how to help him and the types of care available. I would definitely recommend this to anyone. Thank you so much for writing this book.

✓   Thank you for educating us on LBD. I highly recommend this book to anyone who has a loved one diagnosed with LBD and wants to learn about it.

✓   This book opened my eyes and heart in ways that no doctor, nurse, elder expert or shiny pamphlet could do. This book tells it like it is, clearly and calmly, and without holding back about the messy parts.

✓   I am grateful you wrote this book and it will really help me when dealing with the symptoms of LBD in my husband. It touched my heart as it was written with so much empathy, compassion and knowledge. Tough roads ahead are always smoothed if there is a companion at your side and this book is going to be just that through my journey. Thank you for sharing all that you went through so things may be easier for us.

Contents

1. Introduction
2. Dedication
3. Our story - Mum before dementia
4. Dementia - A quick overview
5. Dementia - Young-onset dementia
6. Our story - The warning signs
7. Lewy who - An overview of Lewy body diseases
8. Lewy who - An overview of Parkinson's disease
9. Lewy who - An overview of Lewy body dementias
10. Lewy who - The symptoms of dementia with Lewy bodies
11. Our story - The early symptoms
12. Our story - Getting the diagnosis
13. Lewy who - Diagnosing dementia with Lewy bodies
14. Dementia - Stigma
15. Dementia - Drugs used in dementia
16. Lewy who - Antipsychotic drugs
17. Our story - The descent
18. Dementia - Sundowning
19. Our story - Hospitalisation
20. Our story - Choosing a care home
21. Our story - Rivermead care home
22. Dementia - Time-shift and reminiscence therapy
23. Dementia - Communication
24. Our story - Later stages
25. Lewy who - Stages of Lewy body dementia

26. Dementia - Therapeutic lies
27. Our story - The final journey
28. Dementia - Dysphagia
29. Our story - The end
30. Our story - Timeline
31. Lewy who - The most challenging symptoms
32. Lewy who - Fluctuating cognition
33. Lewy who - Hallucinations
34. Lewy who - Multitasking and problem solving
35. Lewy who - Motor problems
36. Lewy who - Visual perception and illusions
37. Lewy who - Falls in blood pressure & dizziness
38. Lewy who - REM sleep behaviour disorder
39. Dementia - The 7 A's of dementia
40. Our story - The 10 most important things I learnt
41. Lewy who - Important information
42. Just Be Dementia Friendly
43. Final Note
44. References

1. Introduction

Our Mum had dementia with Lewy bodies. Before Mum got ill, I was fairly ignorant about dementia in general, and I had never even heard of dementia with Lewy bodies.

However, I now firmly believe that if at the beginning of Mum's illness, we had known what we know now, then the journey would have been easier for all of us and we would have been able to keep Mum at home for longer than we did.

They say that each person will experience dementia in their own way and that the symptoms and rate of progression will vary from person to person. This makes perfect sense as everyone has their own personality, values and life experiences. But what I didn't appreciate until Mum got ill, is that the type of dementia a person has, will also have a fundamental impact on the earlier symptoms they experience and the care and support they will need. For example, in the early stages of Alzheimer's disease, one of the main symptoms is memory lapses and forgetfulness, whereas for people with dementia with Lewy bodies, day to day memory usually remains fairly intact. However, people with dementia with Lewy bodies often experience hallucinations from early on in the disease whereas with Alzheimer's this doesn't tend to happen until the later stages.

As each type of dementia progresses and more of the brain becomes damaged, the symptoms become more similar. Yet, the impact of the disease in the earlier stages, differ greatly depending on the type of dementia you have. I think it is easiest explained with one simple statement – Same Destination ... Different Journey.

Whilst the campaign to raise awareness has begun, it is important that people understand about the lesser-known types of dementia such as dementia with Lewy bodies. An understanding is crucial in being able to properly describe the symptoms to get an early, accurate diagnosis and to be able to provide relevant care.

It is for this reason that I am now passionate about raising awareness about dementia in general but in particular about dementia with Lewy bodies. It is why I am writing this book, to pass on what I have learnt, to share our story and to highlight the key information you will need if you or someone you love is affected by this horrendous disease.

Although there were three of us who were primarily involved in Mum's journey, this story is written entirely from my perspective and details how Mum's journey impacted and influenced me personally.

Throughout this book, you will learn that there are two types of Lewy body dementias but I have mainly used the classification of dementia with Lewy bodies, as this is the type of dementia that Mum had and the majority of information included relate to the symptoms she experienced.

I would also like to highlight that I am no expert in dementia. Everything in this book is what I have researched following Mum's illness and what I have experienced firsthand with Mum. Chapter 44 includes the websites I have found most useful.

I have split the book into three categories. Firstly, there is our story, which covers everything we went through on our journey with Mum. It covers the highs and the lows and the impact it had on our family life. Secondly, there are a few chapters on dementia, which include information about dementia in general. The third section is specifically dedicated to dementia with Lewy bodies, the type Mum had and in my opinion, the cruellest one of all.

Mum's illness and subsequent death has had a profound impact on my life. Although I know we did the best we possibly could for Mum, with the information we had at the time, I also know that we could have done so much better if we had known all the information included in this book at the start of our journey. I hope it is information that you will find helpful if you end up on a Lewy body dementia journey of your own.

2. Dedication

In Loving Memory of our Mum

Christine Ann Marshall (née Oakley).

<u>A daughter's decree to Lewy body</u>

It was then that you carried me,
throughout the whole of my life,
keeping me safe and away from all strife.

And now that you struggle with everyday things,
I'll make sure your safe from the pain that life brings.
And now that your quality and love of life's gone,
I'll get you the best from each day till you're done.

And as people wonder and as people stare,
as you're talking to things that just are not there.
I will stand beside you and I'll make them see,
if it's real to you, then it's real to me.

And the times that you stumble, the times that you fall,
I'll make sure there's someone to answer your call.
And when you are dizzy, scared and alone,
I'll make sure that kindness and compassion is shown.

When I recently asked you what life had been?
you looked at me sadly and said ordinary.
But I will make sure though the best of you's gone,
that together we create a legacy that's strong.

So as comprehension is the last thing to go,
I hope you can hear me, I pray that you know,
It is now that I carry you.

by Emma Haslegrave

3. Our story: Mum before dementia

Our Mum was born on the 28th May 1942 and was named Christine Ann Oakley.

Her dad was a policeman and was involved in solving a couple of infamous murders in Wakefield, working his way up to the senior rank of Assistant Chief Constable in the Wakefield City Police, as it was then. As a result of his hectic work life, I got the impression that he wasn't around much when Mum was growing up, but never the less she simply adored her dad.

Her Mum was a housewife who was beset with health problems including diabetes, resulting in gangrene, losing both big toes and she also suffered from glaucoma, eventually going blind.

Mum had one older brother, a roguish character who started his career in the Navy but quickly realized he wasn't good with authority. He then moved on to various shady jobs including barman, night club bouncer and general wheeler-dealer. He married three times; his first marriage produced 3 children but ended in divorce. His second marriage was to Lady Julia Montagu, daughter of the Earl of Sandwich. This marriage only lasted 16 months, and following their separation Mum's brother was quoted by the Sun newspaper as saying, "It looks as though our social differences were too great." You don't say! His third and longest marriage was to someone he met in an east end pub, worlds apart from Lady Julia. This marriage produced 2 children.

Mum went to the Girls High School in Wakefield and after deciding on a career in teaching, spent one year as an unqualified assistant before entering Teacher Training College in 1961. Mum went onto become a teacher and spent most of her working life, firstly at Byron First School in Bradford and then Bronte Middle School in Oakworth near Keighley. Mum was passionate about teaching and relished helping kids reach their full potential. While working at Byron First School, which was an inner-city school in a fairly deprived area, Mum used to give up two weeks of her time during the summer holidays and run a summer camp, giving the kids opportunities they would never otherwise have had.

Mum married my Dad and went onto have two children, myself and my younger sister Kate. My Dad was a policeman and an alcoholic, so wasn't around much as we were growing up. As a result Mum, being the only constant, reliable figure in my life, became my world.

Ours was a happy childhood, we were born in an age when kids used to 'play out' and we would spend all our free time out exploring. Looking back now, the amount of freedom we had then seems rather irresponsible but I know it was the 'norm' rather than bad parenting!

I was quite shy growing up, as Mum had been, and I think she overcompensated for this, determined that I wouldn't suffer in the way she had. She would always jump in (perhaps too readily) to fight my battles, and while I was always grateful for her support, it made me all the more dependent on her and probably didn't help me overcome my shyness.

Growing up Dad was always the 'fun' one and Mum more the disciplinarian. However, I realize now, that Dad was actually drunk when he got in the swimming pool fully dressed at my birthday party and that wasn't much 'fun' for Mum.

Mum and Dad eventually divorced when I was around 13 and Mum met and subsequently married Steve, another policeman but infinitely more reliable than Dad. So, as I moved into my teenage years Mum became more relaxed, probably as she didn't have to deal with everything effectively alone, and she became a 'cool' Mum. Me and my friends would pinch Steve's homemade wine and get drunk and I'm sure Mum covered for us, never commenting or condemning.

Mum also loved a drink and a good time and as I got older still Mum and I would frequently go out for a drink and a meal. We would also go and visit my sister, who lived in London at the time, spending the days sightseeing and the evenings in the pub – and late afternoons as well if I'm honest.

I can't remember a time when Mum and I fell out or she became annoyed at me, even when she had every right to be upset (although she must have done when I was younger as I remember getting the odd smack around the legs). Once my partner and I borrowed Mum's beloved campervan and drove it into an underground car park – let's just say the roof of the car park was lower than the roof of the van! Although it was obviously an accident I was still distraught at wrecking Mum's van and was really nervous about ringing her to tell her what had happened. However Mum, as usual, was fabulous that day. She was really concerned that I was so upset and I remember her saying, "Please don't get upset, it's not the end of the world, the main thing is that you're ok." That's how it was with Mum, no matter how bad things seemed, she came along and made everything ok again.

I had always lived within walking distance of Mum and used to see her a couple of times a week but then in 2002, Mum and Steve moved to Filey as Mum had always loved the sea. We used to visit Mum every month until in 2009 we also moved to Filey – never could quite manage to cut the apron strings!

So throughout my life, Mum has been a constant, supportive figure who I have enjoyed spending time with. She has always been, quite simply, my rock.

4. Dementia: A quick overview

Dementia is not a disease in itself. The word dementia is used to describe a group of symptoms including a decline in judgement and understanding, memory loss, confusion and mood changes. There are a number of diseases which cause dementia:

- ✓ Alzheimer's disease is the most common.
- ✓ Vascular dementia.
- ✓ Mixed dementia.
- ✓ Dementia with Lewy bodies.
- ✓ Frontotemporal dementia.
- ✓ Many other rarer forms of dementia.

Most types of dementia are progressive. This means that the structure and chemistry of the brain become increasingly damaged over time. A person's ability to remember, understand, communicate and reason gradually declines.

Each type of dementia has a different cause and affects different parts of the brain, which is why the symptoms in the earlier stages of each disease vary.

Alzheimer's disease is caused as proteins build up in the brain to form structures called plaques and tangles. This leads to the loss of connections between nerve cells, and eventually to the death of nerve cells and loss of brain tissue.

Vascular dementia is caused by reduced blood supply to the brain due to diseased blood vessels.

It is possible to have more than one type of dementia at the same time, known as **mixed dementia**. Alzheimer's is sometimes seen with vascular dementia, the most common form of mixed dementia. Alzheimer's can also be seen with dementia with Lewy bodies. In some cases, a person may have brain changes linked to all 3 conditions – Alzheimer's disease, vascular dementia and dementia with Lewy bodies.

Lewy body dementia is caused by tiny deposits of protein in nerve cells (known as Lewy bodies) and their presence is linked to low levels of important chemical messengers (mainly acetylcholine and dopamine) and to a loss of connections between nerve cells. Over time, there is progressive death of nerve cells and loss of brain tissue.

Frontotemporal dementia is caused when nerve cells in the frontal and/or temporal lobes of the brain die and the pathways that connect them change. There is also some loss of important chemical messengers. Over time, the brain tissue in the frontal and temporal lobes shrinks.

As mentioned, most types of dementia are progressive and will get gradually worse over time, resulting in death. The progression of dementia is broadly categorised into 3 stages:

- ✓ Early (mild) stage - In the early stages of dementia, a person's symptoms will become more noticeable and will start to affect their day-to-day life. However, someone in the early

14

stages of dementia will be able to function independently and should be able to do most things with a little help, or minor adjustments.

✓ Middle (moderate) stage - In the middle stages of dementia the symptoms will become much more obvious and people will start to need more support to help them manage the tasks of daily living.

✓ Late (severe) stage - During the later stages of dementia, most people will become increasingly frail due to the progression of the illness. They will also gradually become dependent on others for all aspects of their care.

Dementia is not a normal part of ageing. However, the brain does get smaller and communication between cells becomes less effective as we get older and some cognitive (thinking) changes happen as a result.

Below is a quick summary of the cognitive changes a person may experience as they get older.

✓ Normal age-related cognitive decline – minor cognitive changes, which are subtle and barely noticeable, that happen as part of normal ageing.

✓ Mild cognitive impairment (MCI) – where someone has problems with their memory and/or thinking skills, which are noticeable to themselves or others but do not have a significant impact on their daily lives.

✓ Dementia – where someone has a set of symptoms which may include memory loss, difficulties with thinking, problem solving or language, which have become severe enough to affect daily life.

Note: Although it is not inevitable, a person with MCI is more likely to develop dementia. In some cases, experts believe MCI is a result of brain changes occurring in the very early stages of dementia. However, in other cases, MCI will turn out to have a different, often treatable cause, such as depression, stress or a physical illness such as a urine infection.

5. Dementia: Young-onset dementia

One of the main risks of developing dementia is age and dementia usually affects people over the age of 65. However, some people develop dementia much younger, which is known as young-onset dementia.

Young-onset dementia, also known as early-onset dementia or working-age dementia, refers to people whose symptoms start before the age of 65. In cases where the symptoms start after the age of 65, it is known as late-onset dementia.

Most people and organisations avoid using the term early-onset dementia to avoid confusion with the early stages of dementia generally.

Although the diseases that cause late-onset dementia are largely the same as young-onset dementia, there are some differences:

- ✓ There is some evidence that young-onset dementia is a more aggressive disease, with the later stage symptoms progressing more quickly.
- ✓ People with young-onset dementia are much more likely to have a rarer form of dementia (around 20% - 25%).
- ✓ Young-onset dementia is also more likely to cause problems with movement, walking, coordination or balance.
- ✓ Young-onset dementia is much more likely, than late-onset dementia, to be hereditary.

Note: In the majority of cases, dementia is not inherited from a family member but is a result of other factors such as age, lifestyle and medical history. In a small number of cases however, dementia is inherited as a result of a faulty gene.

Types of young-onset dementia include:
Young-onset Alzheimer's disease is rare and accounts for up to 5% of all cases (with half of these as a result of familial Alzheimer's disease, see below). Non-familial young-onset Alzheimer's can develop in people who are in their 30's or 40's, but that is extremely rare, with the majority of people in their 50's or early 60's.

Familial Alzheimer's disease is an inherited disease passed down by a faulty gene from an affected parent. Familial Alzheimer's disease usually develops between 50 and 65 years of age, but can be as early as 15. Familial Alzheimer's disease accounts for approximately half the cases of young-onset Alzheimer's disease.

Vascular dementia is caused by reduced blood flow to the brain, often as a result of a stroke or a series of small strokes and is thought to account for 15% - 20% of cases of dementia in the under 65's.

In addition, there is a rare form of vascular dementia caused by faulty genes, known as CADSIL (cerebral autosomal dominant arteriopathy with subcortical infarcts and leukoencephalopathy). CADSIL can be passed down through families and is most common in people aged 30 to 50.

Although **frontotemporal dementia** is one of the less common forms of dementia, it is a significant cause of dementia in younger people. Frontotemporal dementia is most often diagnosed between the ages of 45 and 65. In around a third of people, it can be triggered by a genetic problem known as familial FTD.

Dementia with Lewy bodies accounts for about 5% - 10% of cases of dementia in younger people.

Korsakoff's syndrome, also known as alcohol-related brain damage, is caused by a lack of vitamin B1 (thiamine), often as a result of alcoholism. Korsakoff's syndrome accounts for around 10% of dementia in younger people.

Around 20% - 25% of younger people with dementia are thought to have a **rarer cause** of the condition including:

✓ Progressive supranuclear palsy (PSP) mainly affects people over the age of 60, although it occasionally affects younger people.
✓ Corticobasal degeneration (CBD) mostly develops in adults aged between 50 and 70.
✓ Creutzfeldt-Jakob disease (CJD). There are 4 main types of CJD including an inherited version. The age of onset depends on the type but typically affects younger people.
✓ Niemann-Pick disease type C is one of a group of rare inherited disorders that mainly affects school-age children but can occur at any time, from early infancy to adulthood.

- ✓ Huntington's disease, which is typically inherited from a person's parents, usually appears in a person's 30's or 40's but more rarely appears in adolescence.

6. Our story: The warning signs

I can't remember when we first realized that something wasn't right with Mum, but now with the benefit of hindsight, I realize that something was amiss in June 2009.

That month was my 40th birthday and I remember Mum saying to me, "I'd like to get you a keepsake, if you go buy it, I will give you the money." Normally Mum would have just bought me something or at the very least we would have gone shopping together. Looking back it was as if she knew she should get me something, she wanted to, but just couldn't actually manage to do it herself.

I also remember on my actual birthday, I called around on the way to the pub and asked if she wanted to come for a birthday drink, something she would normally have jumped at. Steve was sawing up a settee that day (don't ask!) and Mum said, "I had better stay and help Steve." At the time I remember thinking how odd it was and feeling faintly offended but at that stage I certainly wasn't thinking dementia.

Much later, my sister also told me that she had tried to arrange a Spa weekend for the three of us for my '40th' but she hadn't been able to pin Mum down with any firm arrangements, which was also out of character as usually Mum would have jumped at the chance of the three of us going away together.

It's funny how I try to think back to when her problems started and can't pinpoint it. In early 2010, Dad's brother died and Mum, Kate and I went to the funeral and I have tried to remember whether her behaviour was unusual. I can't remember anything amiss but Kate can remember that she seemed 'all over the place.'

What I do know is that by October 2011, it was obvious something was wrong, and although we didn't have a diagnosis, we were fairly sure that it was dementia. That month I went to the USA for a fortnight and I remember Mum asking me over and over again, when I was going, where I was going, how long for and when I'd be back.

There are other key incidents that stick in my mind as been significant. I remember one day sat in the garden, and for some reason Mum was trying to convince us that everything was fine when Steve said, "Ok then, who is the current Prime Minister?"

Mum had a think about this for a minute and then replied, "Gordon Brown," when in fact it was David Cameron. Although I can't remember when this conversation took place, David Cameron came to power in May 2010 so it is likely it was around that time.

So there you have it, somewhere between June 2009 and October 2011, we came to the horrifying conclusion that our Mum had dementia. Although at that stage, I don't think I had even heard of dementia with Lewy bodies, so we were thinking it was either Alzheimer's disease or perhaps vascular dementia, as a result of a mild heart attack Mum had in 2005.

Although we are unable to pinpoint exactly when we realized that something was wrong, I do remember that it seemed to happen quickly. One minute she seemed relatively ok (concerns in 2009 and 2010 but only with the benefit of hindsight) and the next she was anything but (shockingly confused by 2011). Obviously, we now know that she had dementia with Lewy bodies, which often has a rapid or acute onset and that's how it seemed with her.

7. Lewy who: An overview of Lewy body diseases

Lewy body diseases are a group of conditions caused by deposits of an abnormal protein called Lewy bodies inside brain cells (named after the doctor Friedrich H Lewy, who discovered them while researching Parkinson's disease). There are 3 types of Lewy body diseases:

Parkinson disease - The main symptoms of Parkinson's are tremor, rigidity and slowness of movement.

Dementia with Lewy bodies - Symptoms include changes in thinking and reasoning, fluctuating cognition, balance problems and muscle rigidity, visual hallucinations, delusions, trouble interpreting visual information, sleep disorders, malfunctions of the autonomic nervous system (the part of the nervous system that regulates bodily functions) and memory loss (but less prominent than in Alzheimer's).

Parkinson's disease dementia - Symptoms include changes in memory, concentration and judgement, trouble interpreting visual information, muffled speech, visual hallucinations, delusions, depression and sleep disturbances.

Together dementia with Lewy bodies and Parkinson's disease dementia are referred to as Lewy body dementias.

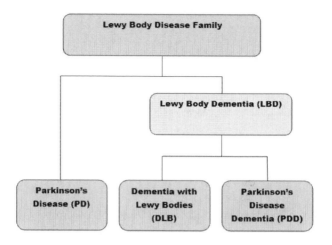

Whether dementia with Lewy bodies or Parkinson's disease dementia is diagnosed will depend on when the cognitive (thinking) impairment appears relative to the Parkinson's disease symptoms (movement).

The diagnosis is dementia with Lewy bodies when:

✓ Dementia symptoms develop first.
✓ When both dementia symptoms and movement symptoms are present at the time of diagnosis.
✓ When dementia symptoms appear within one year after movement symptoms.

The diagnosis is Parkinson's disease dementia when a person is originally diagnosed with Parkinson's and dementia symptoms don't appear until a year or more later.

✓ About one-third of people diagnosed with Parkinson's disease eventually develop dementia (Parkinson's disease dementia). The average time from the onset of Parkinson's to developing dementia is about 10 years.

✓ Similarly, at least two-thirds of people with dementia with Lewy bodies develop movement problems at some point.

✓ Someone aged 50-60 with Lewy bodies in their brain, is more likely to develop Parkinson's disease.

✓ Someone aged 70-80 with Lewy bodies in their brain, is more likely to develop dementia with Lewy bodies.

A significant difference between Parkinson's disease and dementia with Lewy bodies is the location of the Lewy bodies in the brain.

Disease name	Location in the brain	Function controlled	Symptoms
Dementia with Lewy bodies.	Cerebral cortex (outer layer of the brain).	Cognition.	Dementia.
Parkinson's disease.	Substantia nigra (located in the mid brain).	Motor.	Movement Problems.
Parkinson's disease dementia.	Both.	Both.	Both.

In Parkinson's disease, they are found mainly in the substantia nigra which is in the mid-brain, whereas in dementia with Lewy bodies they are more widely distributed throughout the cerebral cortex.

8. Lewy who: An overview of Parkinson's disease

Although this is a book about dementia, I wanted to include this section on Parkinson's disease, as it is a Lewy body disease and people with dementia with Lewy bodies often go on to develop some of the movement and non-movement problems listed below – including Mum.

Parkinson's disease is a progressive neurological condition i.e. it affects the nervous system and gets worse over time. Parkinson's disease is caused by the loss of dopamine producing brain cells and the presence of Lewy bodies in the substantia nigra.

The main symptoms of Parkinson's affect movement and often start on one side of the body first, before affecting both sides.

- ✓ Tremor – shaking is usually one of the first symptoms and affects most people with Parkinson's disease. It usually begins in the hand or arm, is most obvious when at rest, and is reduced when moving or sleeping.
- ✓ Muscle rigidity (stiffness) is a common symptom of Parkinson's disease. This can make it difficult to move limbs.
- ✓ Slowness of movement (bradykinesia) is common in people with Parkinson's disease and can result in them developing a slow shuffling walk.

As different muscles become affected, people with Parkinson's may develop:

- ✓ Problems with their posture and balance – making falls more likely.
- ✓ Speech changes – resulting in their speech becoming quiet, faster, slower or shaky and people may find it harder to understand them.
- ✓ Loss of facial expression – they may smile less, frown more and blink slowly.
- ✓ Small handwriting.

There are also other symptoms that aren't related to movement, including:

- ✓ Mental health problems, such as depression, memory loss, difficulty reasoning and increased anxiety.
- ✓ Bowel and bladder problems such as constipation and the need to urinate often.
- ✓ Problems with swallowing.
- ✓ Excessive production of saliva and drooling.
- ✓ Reduced appetite, leading to weight loss.
- ✓ Impotence.
- ✓ Low blood pressure, causing dizziness on standing.
- ✓ Increased or reduced sweating.
- ✓ Loss of the sense of smell, which may occur years before other symptoms develop.
- ✓ Problems sleeping and tiredness.

Although Parkinson's disease is the most common, there are other neurological diseases that cause problems with movement. As dementia is the umbrella term to describe the symptoms that occur when the brain is affected by diseases such as Alzheimer's, Parkinsonism is the umbrella term used to describe the symptoms of tremors, muscle rigidity and slowness of movement.

Diseases that cause Parkinsonism include:

- ✓ Parkinson's disease (also known as Idiopathic Parkinson's disease) is the most common cause.
- ✓ Multiple system atrophy (MSA).
- ✓ Vascular Parkinsonism.
- ✓ Progressive supranuclear palsy (PSP).
- ✓ Normal pressure hydrocephalus.
- ✓ Drug-induced Parkinsonism.

9. Lewy who: An overview of Lewy body dementias

As mentioned previously there are two types of Lewy body dementias:

- ✓ **Dementia with Lewy bodies** – in which cognitive (thinking) symptoms appear within a year of movement problems.
- ✓ **Parkinson's disease dementia** – in which cognitive symptoms develop more than a year after the onset of movement problems.

Although official statistics state that Lewy body dementias account for 4% of all dementia cases, the actual figure is thought to be much higher, between 15% - 20%, making it the second most common form of dementia behind Alzheimer's disease. There are no brain scans or medical tests that can definitively diagnose Lewy body dementia. Currently, Lewy body dementia can only be diagnosed, with certainty, by a brain autopsy after death – which may account for why it is often misdiagnosed.

Note: See chapter 13 for details on new criteria which can help healthcare professionals give a probable diagnosis of dementia with Lewy bodies.

Difference between dementia with Lewy bodies and Parkinson's disease dementia

The main difference between the two Lewy body dementias, which essentially share the same range of symptoms, is how the disease starts i.e. whether the movement or cognitive problems occur first as detailed above. The other main differences are:

- ✓ In dementia with Lewy bodies, tremor does not occur early and is less severe than in Parkinson's.
- ✓ In dementia with Lewy bodies, problems with the autonomic nervous system are more prominent than in Parkinson's disease dementia.
- ✓ In Parkinson's disease dementia, psychiatric symptoms (e.g. hallucinations, delusions) appear to be less frequent and/or less severe than in dementia with Lewy bodies.
- ✓ Dementia with Lewy bodies may progress more quickly than Parkinson's disease dementia.

Differences between Alzheimer's disease and dementia with Lewy bodies

Alzheimer's is the most common form of dementia and although Alzheimer's and dementia with Lewy bodies have several similarities, there are also some clear differences between the two diseases, which I also wanted to highlight. The main differences are:

- ✓ Memory loss tends to be a more prominent symptom in early Alzheimer's disease than in dementia with Lewy bodies.
- ✓ Movement symptoms are more likely to be an important cause of disability in early dementia with Lewy bodies. Although Alzheimer's can cause problems with walking, balance and

getting around as the disease progresses to moderate and severe stages.

✓ Hallucinations, delusions and misidentification of familiar people (see the section on Capgras syndrome in chapter 41) are significantly more frequent in early stage dementia with Lewy bodies than with Alzheimer's.

✓ Dementia with Lewy bodies patients experience more depression than do Alzheimer's patients.

✓ REM sleep behaviour disorder is more common in early dementia with Lewy bodies than in Alzheimer's disease.

✓ Disruption of the autonomic nervous system, causing a blood pressure drop on standing, dizziness, falls and urinary incontinence is much more common in early dementia with Lewy bodies than in Alzheimer's disease.

✓ Life expectancy is slightly shorter for people with dementia with Lewy bodies than for Alzheimer's patients.

10. Lewy who: The symptoms of dementia with Lewy bodies

The symptoms of dementia with Lewy bodies fall into five categories:

Cognition

The dictionary definition of cognition is *the mental action or process of acquiring knowledge and understanding through thought, experience, and the senses* and people with dementia with Lewy bodies experience the following cognitive changes:

- ✓ Dementia is a primary symptom i.e. a decline in the cognitive abilities that interferes with everyday life.
- ✓ Changes or 'fluctuations' in cognition. The person will swing from a state of alertness to appearing drowsy and/or confused, as well as having a reduced attention span.
- ✓ Recurrent visual hallucinations, such as seeing shapes, colours, people or animals that aren't there or conversing with deceased loved ones.
- ✓ More trouble with complex mental activities, such as multitasking, problem solving and analytical thinking.
- ✓ Problems with visual and spatial perception, such as judging and navigating distances.

Note: Unlike other types of dementia, memory problems may not be evident at first but often arise as the disease progresses.

Motor problems

People with dementia with Lewy bodies experience motor problems (the part of the nervous system involved with movement), similar to Parkinson's including:

- ✓ Slow movement.
- ✓ Shuffling walk.
- ✓ Stiff limbs.
- ✓ Tremors and shaking.
- ✓ Balance problems.
- ✓ Difficulty swallowing.
- ✓ Weak voice.

Autonomic problems

They also experience fluctuations in autonomic processes (the part of the nervous system that regulates key involuntary functions such as breathing, heart rate, digestive processes and body temperature) including:

- ✓ Falls in blood pressure.
- ✓ Changes in body temperature.
- ✓ Urinary difficulties.
- ✓ Constipation.
- ✓ Dizziness.
- ✓ Frequent falls and fainting.
- ✓ Impaired sense of smell.
- ✓ Runny nose.

Sleep disorders

Sleep problems include:

- ✓ REM sleep behaviour disorder – a disorder where you physically move limbs and talk while sleeping (see chapter 38).
- ✓ Insomnia.
- ✓ Excessive daytime sleeping.

Behaviour & mood

Changes in behaviour and mood (psychiatric disturbances) often occur with dementia with Lewy bodies including:

- ✓ Depression.
- ✓ Apathy.
- ✓ Anxiety.
- ✓ Agitation.
- ✓ Delusions.
- ✓ Paranoia.

11. Our story: The early symptoms

So from nowhere, we were dealing with a whole set of symptoms we simply didn't understand. Now I know more about dementia with Lewy bodies, all the symptoms we had to deal with from very early on in Mum's illness, are the classic symptoms of the disease. However, at the time, we had never even heard of it and much of her behaviour was utterly baffling and quite frankly alarming.

Although I will go into her symptoms and what we did to try and manage them in more detail throughout the book, below is a summary of the array of symptoms that we suddenly faced.

- ✓ **Repetitive questions**. This wasn't a big issue with Mum but she easily lost track of the time and was always asking what day it was.
- ✓ **Losing things** (or rather putting them somewhere safe!). We seemed to spend hours looking for things, in particular her glasses and purse.
- ✓ **Unable to recognize her own home.** She used to get very agitated as to why we had sold her house without her permission and was always asking to go home even when she was sat in her own front room.
- ✓ She was very **suspicious**, often accusing us of various things, in particular stealing her purse and selling her house!

✓ **Fluctuating cognition**. One of the key features of dementia with Lewy bodies is that the symptoms vary (fluctuate) widely day by day and even throughout the day. One minute Mum would be okay and then she would suddenly become confused, restless or agitated.

✓ **Short attention span.** Mum would start doing something, quickly lose focus and move onto something else and as a result the house was usually in a state of chaos.

✓ **Dizzy Spells**. Mum would become dizzy when she stood up. Sometimes it would pass quickly but often, if we were out in unfamiliar surroundings, it wouldn't.

✓ **Difficulty with depth/space perception**. She was always bumping into things and going up and down stairs were a particular problem.

✓ **Unable to perform simple tasks.** Mum struggled to perform the most basic tasks, stopped cleaning and cooking, struggled to make a cup of coffee/tea and simply couldn't hang her clothes up in the wardrobe.

✓ **Visual hallucinations**. Another key feature of dementia with Lewy bodies, you would often find Mum chatting away to someone/thing and most mornings she would get incredibly flustered, insisting she needed to take a register of all the children in the kitchen.

✓ **Illusions.** Mum would incorrectly see a real object, such as a cushion, as something else, such as a cat, so you would often find her sat stroking and talking to a cushion.

✓ **Delusions**. Possibly as a result of her hallucinations, Mum was convinced that there were a group of strangers living on the ground floor, which in turn strengthened her conviction that it wasn't her house.

✓ **Shuffling walk.** In the early stages, this only tended to be noticeable if she was tired or stressed. She would lean forward and take little shuffling steps, often falling as a result.

✓ **Agitation**. Mum would become highly restless and agitated – often suddenly. It would often start with questions as to why we had sold the house and no amount of reassurance that it was her house would settle her. This anxiety always increased around 4 pm, a phenomenon known as 'sundowning' (see chapter 18).

12. Our story: Getting the diagnosis

Once we realized that something was wrong with Mum, and we were fairly sure it was dementia, we were keen to get a diagnosis. Mainly so that Mum could receive medication to help slow the progression of the disease, but also for any medication that could help with her anxiety.

One of the main obstacles to getting a diagnosis was Mums utter refusal to accept there was a problem or to discuss it in any way. I think the main issue was that Mum herself had a very ignorant and stigmatized view of dementia. She insisted that she was far too intelligent to have dementia and that there was no way we were carting her off to the 'loony bin' (her words not mine).

I suppose Mum grew up in an era where there was significant stigma attached to dementia. Although this is starting to change I believe it is imperative that work continues to remove the stigma from dementia. Not only to ensure that people receive more help and understanding in the community but also to help them accept their illness without fear or embarrassment. Throughout Mum's illness, the very word dementia would send her into an episode of either extreme anger or sadness.

Mum's attitude really didn't help us in getting a diagnosis. She absolutely refused to take a memory test, which is what the doctor was insisting needed to happen, so we were stuck in a 'catch 22' situation. We eventually managed to get Mum to agree to the test by using good old fashioned emotional blackmail, which we hated doing but didn't feel we had much choice. By this point, she was struggling with some of the most basic day to day tasks and was frequently hallucinating, which we found very difficult to deal with.

Imagine our surprise and Mum's elation when we were told that she had passed the memory test and the doctor concluded that Mum was simply depressed. With dementia with Lewy bodies, memory is largely intact in the earlier stages of the disease, which could account for why she seemed to sail through the test. In addition, fluctuating cognition can mean that people with dementia with Lewy bodies have periods of near-normal functioning, and although I can't remember, Mum must have been having a good day when she took the test.

So we struggled on, with Mum more adamant than ever there wasn't a problem. However, there came a point where we could ignore it no longer so I made some more calls to the doctor who just kept saying she needed to take another memory test.

Eventually, I booked an appointment for myself but once there ambushed him about Mum. When he once again raised the issue of a memory test, I asked him what the next steps would be if she had taken and failed the test. He said he would then refer Mum to a specialist but couldn't because he wasn't satisfied there was a problem. Following my refusal to leave the surgery until he agreed to a referral, he reluctantly agreed that if I could get Mum to an appointment with him he would ask some general questions to try and assess her.

So in January 2012, we told Mum she needed to visit the surgery for a blood test result. I went with her and the doctor casually started to ask her some general questions. I am sure he was still of the impression she had depression and was just 'humouring me' so when Mum started off by answering all his questions correctly I could have died – the conversation went as follows:

Doctor - "Can you tell me what day it is?"
Mum - "Tuesday," (which was correct).
Doctor - "Date?"
Mum - "18th," (correct).
Doctor - "Month?"
Mum - "January," (correct).

At this point, the doctor looked at me obviously thinking, I told you there wasn't a problem and I am considering reporting you for elder abuse. I returned a look to say, I am telling you there is a problem and if you continue, she will slip up because she can't maintain this for long. So with an exaggerated sigh the doctor asked, "Year?"

Mum - "Erm, I'm not sure."
Doctor - "As it is a new year, it will be understandable if you are out by a year."
Mum - "No sorry I don't know."

After this, she completely fell apart and couldn't tell him what she had eaten for dinner 30 minutes earlier.

Mum looked so sad and small that day and I remember feeling both deep sadness and utter relief.

But we got the referral to Cross Lane, a psychiatric hospital in Scarborough. The day we first went there with Mum was another traumatic day I will never forget. Mum was still insisting there was nothing wrong with her and became very upset and agitated. We all had a chat with a consultant psychiatrist and Mum was so upset she had to be taken off for a walk. We updated the doctor on all the symptoms Mum was experiencing and he agreed it sounded very much like dementia.

A brain scan was scheduled which terrified Mum and over the coming weeks, until the scan date, Mum was highly agitated and would ask over and over what the scan entailed. For some reason she had got it into her head that it would involve water and she wanted to know if she would need to wear her swimming costume. Each time I went over what would happen and reassured her that there was no water involved, that they were simply going to take some pictures of her head and that it wouldn't hurt in any way. She would eventually calm down but within a couple of hours she would get upset and we would go through the whole process again.

Mum became so anxious that we arranged for the doctor to prescribe some sedatives for the actual day of the scan, as we were concerned that she would simply refuse to go through with it unless we could calm her down.

On the day of the scan Mum was highly agitated so we gave her the sedative. This seemed to do the trick as she happily came to the hospital – well maybe not happily but she came – disappeared off for her scan and then came back and said, "Right are we off then?" We were absolutely astounded and I remember I went off to check that she had actually had the scan because she was so calm about it.

A further visit to Cross Lane was scheduled for the results of the scan and we were told that Mum had vascular dementia, mixed with Alzheimer's disease, as a result of a minor heart attack that she had in 2005. It was March 2012.

At that point some dementia medication was prescribed along with medication to help with her anxiety. We were assigned a consultant psychiatrist, a community psychiatric nurse (CPN) and an approved social worker (ASW), all of whom provided invaluable support over the coming months.

Following the diagnosis, I remember feeling utter relief. Not only because we finally had confirmed what we had suspected for months but also because we were no longer dealing with it alone, as by now we were really struggling to cope.

13. Lewy Who: Diagnosing dementia with Lewy bodies

As mentioned previously there is no way of definitively diagnosing dementia with Lewy bodies, which can only be done with certainty by a brain autopsy after death. As a result, dementia with Lewy bodies is often misdiagnosed.

However in June 2017, the *International Dementia with Lewy Bodies Consortium* published updated diagnostic criteria, called the *Consensus Guidelines* to help add greater weight to a probable/possible diagnosis.

In the guidelines, the symptoms, which are described as clinical features, are categorised as either central/core or supportive.

The **central clinical feature** (symptom) is dementia and this must be present for a diagnosis of dementia with Lewy bodies i.e. a decline in the cognitive (thinking) abilities that interferes with everyday life.

There are four **core clinical features,** listed below. If 2 or more of these symptoms are present then a probable diagnosis can be made. If only 1 is present then a possible diagnosis can be made.

- ✓ Fluctuating cognition (awareness and concentration).
- ✓ Recurrent visual hallucinations, such as seeing shapes, colours, people, or animals that aren't there.

- ✓ REM sleep behaviour disorder, which often presents years before the onset of dementia.
- ✓ Parkinsonism (problems with movement).

Note: Fluctuating cognition and visual hallucinations detected early in the progression of dementia with Lewy bodies (as is often the case) can help differentiate from Alzheimer's disease, where they do not tend to appear until the later stages.

In addition REM sleep behaviour disorder is highly associated with Lewy body disorders but not Alzheimer's disease.

There are also a number of **supportive clinical features** which make a diagnosis more likely, as follows:

- ✓ Severe sensitivity to antipsychotic drugs.
- ✓ Postural instability (poor balance).
- ✓ Repeated falls.
- ✓ Syncope (fainting).
- ✓ Autonomic dysfunction e.g. constipation, falls in blood pressure, urinary incontinence.
- ✓ Hypersomnia (excessive day time sleeping).
- ✓ Hyposmia (reduced ability to smell and to detect odours).
- ✓ Other types of hallucinations i.e. auditory.
- ✓ Delusions.
- ✓ Mood changes i.e. apathy, anxiety and depression.

The guidelines also include 2 indicative and 2 supportive diagnostic bio-markers (e.g. brain scans to detect biological signs of disease). I haven't included the bio-markers here as they are very technical and therefore fairly meaningless to most people – including me. However bio-markers help support the diagnosis of dementia with Lewy bodies. In cases where only 1 core clinical feature is present but 1 indicative bio-marker is also present then a probable diagnosis can be given. If 1 or more indicative bio-marker are present with no core clinical features then a possible diagnosis can be made.

This list would have been really useful to us when we were trying to obtain a diagnosis, as Mum was experiencing the central clinical feature of dementia, all 4 core clinical features in addition to many of the supportive clinical features.

14. Dementia: Stigma

I have included a chapter on stigma because Mum herself had a very stigmatized view of dementia and it definitely prevented her from acknowledging her symptoms and obtaining the help we all needed.

The Oxford dictionary definition of stigma is *a mark of disgrace associated with a particular circumstance, quality, or person.* The Collins dictionary states *if something has a stigma attached to it, people think it is something to be ashamed of.* It's hard to believe that these statements could apply to people living with dementia but there is still a great deal of stigma surrounding the disease and many people often feel ashamed of their diagnosis – including Mum.

There are many reasons why dementia is still so stigmatized, from a lack of public awareness and low levels of understanding through to fear. Most of us fear dementia. And the brutal truth is, that we fear dementia because the public perception is that people with dementia end up as 'empty shells' unable to recognize anyone and completely dependent on others for all aspects of daily living.

There is no doubt that dementia is a horrible disease that strips away memories. Not only memories of loved ones, of a life lived but it also takes our memory of how to do things. Eventually, it takes away the ability to live independently or communicate effectively.

However, throughout Mum's illness I have come to understand that while someone in the later stages of dementia will need help with most aspects of daily living, if the relevant understanding, care and support is in place, they can still do some things for themselves, still participate in the things they enjoy, still maintain their dignity.

Unfortunately, the stigma of dementia is a self-perpetuating problem. Nobody wants to discuss the reality of the later stages of the disease because they fear it. However, if we don't discuss it, we will never improve people's understanding of what can be done to help and support people to live as well as they can with dementia. We will never remove the fear or the stigma. So below is my view on some of the reasons why there is still such a stigma associated with dementia.

The **association of mental illness and lunatic asylums** - The stigma attached to dementia also applies to all types of mental illnesses. Until fairly recently 'lunatic asylums' were commonplace and they were where people with any type of mental illness, including dementia, went if they needed care. The image that lunatic asylums create is one of people in straight-jackets, electric shock treatments and other barbaric practices. So while thankfully these places no longer exist, to Mum's generation, they were the only places available to people with mental health issues and they still remain very vivid in their imaginations.

Negative terminology - Until recently, many of the symptoms of dementia and the associated behaviours were described in negative terms. Words such as 'wandering' used to describe someone who does a lot of walking, suggests 'aimless/thoughtless wandering' and can add to the stigmatized view that people with dementia have no purpose. The term 'challenging behaviours' used to describe behaviours such as aggression or restlessness adds to the stigmatized view that people with dementia are often difficult and unreasonable.

Thankfully things are starting to change and people are encouraged to simply say 'walking about' and 'changes in behaviour' in a step to reduce stigma.

Behavioural changes - People with dementia can sometimes become aggressive, argumentative or difficult, even though it was never in their nature to do so before they became ill. Because someone with dementia is no longer able to apply rational thought, any out of character behaviour becomes more difficult to resolve, making people uncomfortable and/or embarrassed.

However, try and remember that there is nearly always a reason behind changes in behaviour, such as fear, embarrassment, pain or hunger. A reason that they are no longer able to communicate, causing frustration. Try and get to the root cause of the problem and look out for common triggers that may help you understand what is wrong. Avoid confrontation and if necessary use distraction techniques.

Memory Loss - Most people associate memory loss as one of the main features of dementia and forgetting our loved ones is probably one of the things about dementia that we fear the most. Together with the fear that if we forget them, they will stop visiting, hiding behind the 'what's the point if they don't even recognize me' excuse.

But although Mum often forgot my name and our relationship to each other, I always felt that she recognized me as someone she knew and loved. I learnt not to get too hung up on what she called me and instead cherished the lovely smile I used to get on arrival. So if you remain a constant presence in your loved ones life, you may find that one of the things you fear the most…never happens.

Communication - People with dementia struggle to communicate as the disease progresses. Some have fluent speech but without meaning, while others have little or no speech.

The struggle to communicate leads to the perception that people with dementia have nothing meaningful to say. As a result, people with dementia are often dismissed, ignored or overlooked. This can lead to a loss of confidence and reduced well being, making them more likely to withdraw from social interaction, perpetuating the 'empty shell' perception.

But in my experience, people with dementia still have thoughts and opinions and we must find ways to help them express themselves. Never talk over or through someone as though they are not there and don't be embarrassed if you are holding a conversation which makes no sense. Like everyone, people with dementia like to talk and feel as though they are been listened to.

Vulnerability - As dementia progresses people start to need more help with the tasks of daily living. As a result, they lose control of the most basic life choices, such as what to eat and when.

This is another aspect of dementia that people fear, that they will become completely reliant on others. They fear that people may take advantage, or worse still, that they may be mistreated. Personally, Mum's vulnerability was one of the things that scared me the most, that she would be mistreated and wouldn't be able to stand up for herself or raise the alarm.

But the only way to reduce the risk of this happening is to raise awareness so people can better understand the symptoms of dementia and how to manage them.

Personal hygiene - People living with dementia do find it more and more difficult to maintain their personal hygiene. This can lead to people looking more unkempt than usual, which some people find uncomfortable and adds to the stigma that people with dementia no longer care about their appearance.

But it's not necessarily that they no longer care. There are many reasons why personal hygiene becomes more difficult, including a lack of awareness of the last time they took a bath (or the need to) through to being unable to get into/out of the bath. It is also likely that they will need help with bathing which can cause embarrassment.

Raising awareness about the difficulties of personal hygiene for someone living with dementia is crucial, so allowances can be made, relieving pressure on both the person living with dementia and their carers.

Toileting - It is inevitable that people in the later stages of dementia will need help with toileting and in the very advanced stages, when mobility becomes a problem, disposable underwear is sometimes used as a precaution against accidents.

I remember once, towards the end of her life, Mum needed the toilet and I asked a member of staff in the care home where she lived to help me take her to the bathroom. He replied, "There is no need, she is wearing …" I stopped him mid-sentence and after giving him a piece of my mind I made him help me take Mum to the bathroom. I was livid that day because in my experience, even in the advanced stages, people would still prefer to use the toilet albeit with support. And sadly when people aren't given assistance and accidents happen, it is often not the fault of the person with dementia, even though they are the ones who have to live with the stigma.

The stigma of dementia has a significant impact not only on those living with dementia but also their families. Stigma also makes us all fear dementia more than any other disease. Below is how stigma impacts on those living with dementia.

- ✓ Stigma stops people from acknowledging their symptoms.
- ✓ Makes people more reluctant to obtain an early diagnosis (or any diagnosis at all).
- ✓ Without a diagnosis, it limits access to available treatments.
- ✓ Stops people from obtaining the help and support they need.
- ✓ Prevents planning for the future, including where they would like to live in the later stages of the disease.
- ✓ Stops people from participating in clinical trials, needed to improve the lives of those living with dementia and ultimately find a cure.
- ✓ Results in a loss of friendships/changes in relationships.
- ✓ Causes a loss of confidence and reduced well being.

When stigma affects the families of those living with dementia, particularly the primary caregiver, it is known as stigma by association. Examples of stigma by association that family caregivers may experience include:

- ✓ Embarrassment - Family and friends may find it difficult to deal with some of the more challenging symptoms of dementia such as aggressive behaviour or incontinence.
- ✓ Isolation - This can lead to isolation as carers also become excluded, as other family members and friends try to avoid social interaction with those living with dementia.
- ✓ Fear - Carers may worry that a lack of personal hygiene may be mistaken for neglect.
- ✓ Carers and other family members may also struggle with feelings of shame, guilt and anger resulting in increased feelings of caregiver burden.

Sadly throughout Mum's illness, I came across many examples of stigma including:

- ✓ People talking to her like she was a three year old or talking over or through her like she wasn't there.
- ✓ Friends who slowly drifted away and stopped visiting.
- ✓ People commenting because Mum hadn't washed her hair or her clothing wasn't coordinated.
- ✓ People who commented that they were surprised that Mum had dementia because she was a well-educated teacher!
- ✓ In the later stages of the illness, when Mum did struggle to communicate effectively, I had more than one person say, "But your Mum has

effectively gone now." Well she hadn't gone but it demonstrates how some people view the quality and value of the life of those living with dementia.

I also saw the impact that stigma had on Mum and it is one of the reasons why I am so passionate about raising awareness. Nobody should stigmatize dementia because anyone of us could get the condition, it doesn't care about intelligence or strength of character. And it is fair to say that if you don't develop dementia, it is almost certain that someone you know will.

15. Dementia: Drugs used in dementia

Most dementias are progressive, so the symptoms will gradually get worse over time. Although there is no cure, there are drugs available for the treatment of progressive dementia, which may help some people.

The type of drugs used fall into two categories:

- ✓ Dementia drugs which may temporarily slow the progression of the disease and improve the symptoms of dementia such as memory and concentration.
- ✓ Behavioural and psychological drugs which are used to treat the associated symptoms of dementia such as depression and sleep disturbances.

The two most commonly prescribed **dementia drugs** are a) cholinesterase inhibitors and b) memantine.

a) Cholinesterase inhibitors work by boosting levels of a chemical called acetylcholine, involved in nerve cell communication. These drugs work to temporarily improve or stabilize the symptoms of dementia.

The three types of cholinesterase inhibitors currently available are:

- ✓ Donepezil also known as Aricept.
- ✓ Rivastigmine also known as Exelon.
- ✓ Galantamine also known as Razadyne (previously Reminyl).

Although each type of drug works in the same way, some people respond to one type better than others and may experience fewer side effects. Benefits include improvements in thinking, memory and concentration.

These drugs are used to treat people with mild to moderate Alzheimer's although doctors may continue to prescribe one of these drugs for longer if they believe it is still having a beneficial effect. Donepezil is also used to treat more severe Alzheimer's.

Cholinesterase inhibitors may also be helpful for people with both Alzheimer's and vascular dementia (mixed dementia) and are used to help improve some of the symptoms of dementia with Lewy bodies, including thinking skills and visual hallucinations.

The most common side effects of cholinesterase inhibitors are sickness, diarrhea, having trouble sleeping, muscle cramps, and tiredness. These effects are often mild and usually only temporary. Not everyone will experience side effects.

b) Memantine, also known as Namenda, regulates the activity of glutamate, another chemical messenger involved in brain functions such as learning and memory.

Although they don't work for everyone, memantine is recommended as an option for people with severe Alzheimer's disease, and for people with moderate Alzheimer's if cholinesterase inhibitors don't help or are not suitable. It works to temporarily slow down the progression of symptoms and may also help with agitation or aggression, both more common in the later stages of the disease. Memantine is currently only recommended for people with Alzheimer's disease.

The most common side effects of memantine are headaches, dizziness, drowsiness and constipation, although these effects are usually only temporary.

There are a number of **behavioural and psychological drugs** used to alleviate the symptoms of dementia including:

- ✓ Antidepressants can be used to treat depression.
- ✓ Sleeping tablets can help with sleep disturbances.
- ✓ Antipsychotic drugs (also known as neuroleptics and major tranquillizers) can be prescribed for some of the behavioural and psychological symptoms in dementia.

Note: Although antipsychotic drugs can eliminate or reduce the intensity of psychotic symptoms such as delusions and hallucinations and can have a calming effect, work is underway to reduce the use of antipsychotic drugs in dementia care. This is because they are linked to serious side effects, only have a moderate short term benefit and do not address the underlying causes of behaviours such as agitation or aggression.

Mum was prescribed Aricept, to try and improve her dementia symptoms and help reduce anxiety. She was also prescribed Sertraline which is an anti-depressant used to treat depression, panic attacks and anxiety.

16. Lewy who: Antipsychotic drugs

People with a Lewy body dementia may have severe reactions to, or side effects from neuroleptics, also known as antipsychotics. Neuroleptics are medications used to treat delusions, hallucination or agitation which are all common symptoms of Lewy body dementias.

Severe neuroleptic sensitivity affects up to 50% of the Lewy body dementia patients who are treated with traditional antipsychotic medications.

These side effects include:

- ✓ Worsening confusion.
- ✓ Impaired consciousness.
- ✓ Worsening autonomic problems, such as a drop in blood pressure.
- ✓ Worsened Parkinsonism.
- ✓ Symptoms resembling neuroleptic malignant syndrome (NMS), which can be fatal. (NMS causes severe fever, muscle rigidity and breakdown that can lead to kidney failure).

I remember the day that Mum's consultant psychiatrist changed her diagnosis from mixed dementia to dementia with Lewy bodies. He explained a little bit about the disease and how her behaviour fit with the common symptoms. He then went onto tell us about the importance of telling any medical staff that Mum had dementia with Lewy bodies and that antipsychotic drugs could be harmful. He was so adamant that we needed to do this that it immediately stuck in my mind, although I remember thinking at the time but shouldn't they already know that.

Over the coming years, Mum was admitted to hospital on a number of occasions and as instructed I always made sure that the staff were made aware of her condition and that antipsychotic drugs may be harmful. Turns out he was right to insist because every single person I told said, "I didn't know that."

So always make sure that if a person with a Lewy body dementia is taken to hospital, that the staff are made aware of their condition and that antipsychotic drugs may be harmful. Never assume that medical staff will know.

17. Our story: The descent

Once Mum had been diagnosed and had started a course of medication, we were naively hoping that the medication would calm her but it didn't happen and her behaviour deteriorated. Further changes were made to the medication dosage and the time the medication was administered to try and combat the 'sundowning' effect (see chapter 18).

By this stage Mum was highly agitated. She was hallucinating often and was convinced that there was a strange family living in her home. She was also adamant that her home wasn't her own and that we had sold her house without her permission. At this stage we were still trying to convince Mum that there wasn't anyone else in the house and that she was 'seeing things,' which obviously she was but her hallucinations were very real to her. As a result, Mum became paranoid and delusional, convinced everyone was out to trick her into thinking she was going mad.

Mum also became quite secretive and would hide things in case of an emergency. Of course she could never then remember where she had hidden them and would often accuse us of stealing her purse or whatever she had hidden. At this time we were spending at least an hour a day searching for things that had been put somewhere safe. Sometimes things would go missing for days and we would then find the hairdryer under the duvet cover in the spare bedroom, for example.

In addition Mum was always very restless, but it was a struggle to find things to occupy her, as she was simply unable to do the things she had once enjoyed like reading or gardening. She would fixate on something like cleaning all the brassware. So we would go out and buy some Brasso and set her off polishing, but within 5 minutes she would lose interest and move onto something else. As a result, the house was in a constant state of chaos with tasks Mum had started and never finished.

Dressing, bathing and personal hygiene also became a problem from early on. Before her illness, Mum had loved nothing more than soaking in the bath, listening to an audiobook, but she quickly became unwilling to take a bath or shower. Part of the problem was that she struggled to get into and out of the bath and she certainly couldn't do it unaided. Getting Mum dressed was also a problem, partly because she insisted that she didn't need any help, when in fact she did. As a result, Mum was no longer as smart as she once had been and it was very frustrating and upsetting for me when people used to comment. People need to understand the challenges of personal hygiene for someone suffering from dementia and make allowances. From our perspective, it really was the least of our worries if Mum hadn't washed her hair for a few days.

We were very lucky that the consultant psychiatrist appointed to Mum knew a fair bit about dementia with Lewy bodies (it was a different psychiatrist to the one who had given us the initial diagnosis). Following a home visit where he observed her behaviour (she was hallucinating and talking to 'someone'); he asked us various questions and changed the diagnosis in late 2012/early 2013.

Although a key feature of dementia with Lewy bodies is fluctuating cognition, things such as changing medication, physical illness and stress will cause symptoms and behaviour to deteriorate dramatically (see chapter 41). I now think that it is likely that some of the things we were doing to try and help Mum, were in fact making her condition worse. Her medication was constantly been tinkered with and she wasn't eating or drinking much by this point so was probably dehydrated. We were always trying to reassure her that there wasn't anybody else living in the house, something you should avoid doing, as her hallucinations were very real to her. We were also trying to keep Mum engaged in the things she used to enjoy such as helping with the cooking, things that were simply beyond her, causing frustration and embarrassment. In hindsight, everything we were doing was adding pressure to a system that was simply unable to cope.

By now her behaviour was what I can only describe as manic, and we were all beyond stressed. Mum was agitated for much of the day and seemed afraid in her own home. She would often get up and rush out of the house suddenly and if we weren't quick enough to stop her, she was gone and we would spend hours trying to find her. Usually, when we did manage to track her down she would be confused, frightened and distressed.

For a while we tried locking the door but this caused real anger and she would end up kicking the door and banging her head against it. So we were left in a situation where she really couldn't be left alone, even for a few minutes.

It is really difficult to put into words how stressful, upsetting, isolating and soul-destroying it is to see the person you love the most so agitated and distressed, especially when nobody seems to be able to help.

By mid 2013, we were in regular contact with the community psychiatric nurse (CPN), as we were really struggling to cope. They did come up with some practical suggestions, like getting pressure mats on the doors so we would know if she had left the house and arranging for some bath handles to help with bathing. In addition, the psychiatrist was still tinkering with her medication to try and improve her agitation levels and general confusion.

By this stage, Mum refused to stay in the house and soon as she got up in a morning she would be out the door to go 'home.' We spent hours literally wandering the streets with her until she reached the point of exhaustion and we could take her home where she would sleep for a couple of hours.

She also started approaching people in the street asking for help as she believed she was being followed. One evening Mum had left the house in a state and Steve had followed at a safe distance to make sure she was safe (as we were advised to do). Mum had knocked on a door down the road and advised the man who answered that she was being followed and was scared. Initially Mum could seem quite plausible and the man confronted Steve. Luckily as Steve tried to explain the situation it became apparent that Mum was confused and the situation was diffused but things were starting to spiral out of control.

Following yet another emergency call to the CPN, it was agreed with a heavy heart that she needed to be hospitalised whilst they tried to get her medication combination right in a safe and secure environment, as she had become a danger to herself and potentially others.

18. Dementia: Sundowning

Often people with dementia become more confused and/or agitated in the late afternoon and evening. This is known as sundowning as these changes in behaviour occur as the sun goes down. Sundowning is more common in people who are in the mid and late stages of dementia, although Mum suffered from sundowning from quite early on in her illness.

While Mum was at home she would start to get agitated at around 4 pm every day (she may have continued to suffer from sundowning when she was in hospital and the care home but I always tended to visit mornings and stay until early afternoon). This was one of the symptoms that we found particularly difficult to manage; her main symptoms were agitation and restlessness. The only thing that seemed to calm Mum down was going for a walk, which we would do for a couple of hours until Mum was literally tired out and she would then settle a little.

What are the symptoms?
People who are suffering from sundowning may experience:

- ✓ An increase in general confusion.
- ✓ Increased agitation (they may become upset or anxious).
- ✓ They may become more restless.
- ✓ Increased irritability.
- ✓ Disorientation.

✓ They may become more demanding.
✓ Become more suspicious.
✓ Experience mood swings.
✓ Sundowning can also result in an increase in pacing, tremors and/or hallucinations.

What is the cause?
Doctors aren't sure why sundowning happens but many people who experience it have trouble sleeping at night. In turn, fatigue (and end of day exhaustion) is a common cause, other factors may include:

✓ An upset in the internal body clock, causing a biological mix-up between day and night.
✓ As dusk falls, a decrease in lighting and increased shadows, can cause people with dementia to misinterpret what they see and as a result become confused and afraid.
✓ People with dementia may simply be reacting to signs of tiredness and frustration from caregivers who are exhausted from their day.

What can be done to reduce the impact?
It is important that you don't just attribute out of character behaviours to sundowning and overlook other factors which may be causing the behaviour, such as someone struggling to communicate an underlying problem. Firstly, look at and address any other potential reasons why someone is behaving out of character, such as hunger or thirst.

In addition, any underlying illness, such as a urinary tract infection, may worsen sundowning behaviour so check with their doctor if you suspect this may be the case.

Other actions to reduce sundowning include:

- ✓ Regulate sleep. Too much sleep during the day will result in disturbed sleep at night.
- ✓ An early afternoon rest, however, can be beneficial as fatigue can make sundowning worse.
- ✓ Keep rooms well-lit after dusk. This reduces shadows, distracts from the fact that it's dark outside and can help to enhance mood.
- ✓ If there's a window, allow for light exposure in the morning as this can help set the internal body clock.
- ✓ Encourage an active day.
- ✓ Keep a daily routine. Set regular times for waking up, meals, and going to sleep.
- ✓ Try to schedule appointments, outings, visits, and bath time earlier in the day, when they are less tired.
- ✓ Adjust eating patterns, as large meals late in the day can increase agitation and disturb sleep, especially if caffeine or alcohol is consumed.
- ✓ Only do activities that are simple and calming in the afternoon and evening. Things that are too challenging or unusual will increase frustration and stress and add to their confusion and irritability.

✓ In the evening, try to reduce loud background noise. Consider TV viewing carefully; avoid things that are too loud or violent.

✓ Try to be more patient and kind during these hours.

19. Our story: Hospitalisation

I will never forget the day we took Mum to Cross Lane Hospital in Scarborough in August 2013, the worst day of my life at that point. My sister and I took her and because she would never have willingly agreed to go, we told her we were going to the chemist to sort out her tablets. She trustingly came along, like a lamb to the slaughter, and although we didn't know it at the time, she would never return home. Mum was placed on the Rowan Lea ward at Cross Lane, an acute inpatient service for older people.

Mum was beyond distraught that day, as were my sister and I. I remember Mum was sat in a chair with her head in her hands rocking while a team of people asked us loads of questions we could barely answer as we were crying so much. They eventually took Mum off for a walk and after we had finished answering questions we went to find Mum who was frantically trying to find us and the way out. I remember her begging us to take her home and I felt a physical pain in my chest, it was so upsetting. Mum eventually wore herself out and we took her to her room where she fell asleep and we left.

The following day when we went to visit, Mum seemed almost catatonic, barely speaking or moving, which was as upsetting as seeing her so distressed the previous day. I remember wondering whether they had basically 'drugged her up to the eyeballs' but I think it was just her body resting from the previous day's ordeal.

However, I remember leaving that day and saying, "What have we done?"

Mum has always hated doctors, hospitals and especially dentists (out of all rationale proportion), and her time at Cross Lane was not a happy one. Although Mum was in hospital to try and get her medication right, to reduce her agitation and anxiety, I have to say that the environment was not conducive to achieving that result. There were no carpets and all the doors were heavy so there always seemed to be doors slamming and noise which reverberated around the place.

The bedrooms were through a locked door and sometimes if a patient was particularly distressed, they would be allowed into this area, which in theory was quieter. I remember once when I arrived and Mum was nowhere to be seen and I was told she was in the 'bedroom corridor.' When I eventually found her, she was on her own sobbing uncontrollably. The laundry room was in this area, and a member of staff was in and out and each time the door would slam and Mum would jump out of her skin, making her more and more agitated and distressed. I remember sitting with Mum who just kept asking over and over again, "What have I done wrong, why can't I come home?" Another heartbreaking day that will stay with me forever. I finally managed to calm her down, when the laundry room door slammed again and I am sorry to say I 'lost it' with the member of staff concerned. This outburst seemed to cheer Mum up a bit though, so every cloud!

Another problem was that Cross Lane was a hospital and there was no disguising that fact. Mum had to undergo daily tests, such as blood pressure and temperature checks, which used to really distress and upset her. In addition, as the ward was for acute cases, it seemed that everyone was either highly agitated or catatonic. There was one chap in particular who used to literally bounce off the walls. He would be highly agitated and would charge around the place banging into things and shouting obscenities. I have to say that I was a bit wary of him but when he started on one of his rampages Mum would tell him off, take his hand and walk with him until he calmed down.

Finally Mum did seem to settle down and improve and once she stopped being quite so anxious she put her mind to other things. One day I arrived and the head nurse pulled me to one side to tell me she had some 'serious news.' I remember feeling panic until I spotted Mum, who seemed fine, so I followed the nurse into her office to receive this 'news.' "I am sorry to tell you that your Mum escaped as far as the car park yesterday," she said to me seriously. As Cross Lane is a secure unit with two locked doors, a push-button door (which may as well be locked to a dementia patient) and a receptionist, this was in my book, a fairly amazing feat and I think I laughed. The nurse went onto tell me that it wasn't funny – maybe not, but it is impressive – and that Mum had not only done it once, but she had managed it twice. In addition, she had taught others how to do it, as another chap had managed to get through one of the doors as well. As a result, the whole ward had been put

in lockdown, the door engineer had been called out and
Mum had been put under 24-hour surveillance –
something she did not take kindly to! While obviously,
it could have been very serious if Mum had got further
than the car park (only foiled when she was spotted by a
doctor) as she hadn't, I just felt very proud – although I
didn't tell the nurse that who really didn't seem to see
the funny side at all!

It seemed that around this time, Mum spent much of her
time trying to escape and as a result, she was eventually
sectioned under section 3 of the Mental Health Act,
something else she would have hated if she had been
well enough to realize what was happening.

Although her time at Cross Lane was difficult, I do have
some fond memories of this time as well. There is a
garden walk in the grounds of the hospital where we
used to go for a walk and as Mum's treatment
progressed and she improved, I got agreement to take
Mum down to the seafront at Scarborough. We used to
walk on the front and then call at a café for coffee,
happy times I will always cherish.

Earlier on in her stay, when Mum was still agitated, I
would often get a call from a nurse asking me to speak
to Mum as she was upset, in the hope that I would be
able to calm her down. One day I got a call from Cross
Lane, so I answered expecting a nurse but it was Mum.
"Hello love," she said. We then chatted for a while (I
can't remember what about now) and then she said, "I
have to go now, bye love." I remember putting the

phone down and bursting into tears it was so unexpected. The next time I visited I asked a nurse about it and she told me that Mum had knocked on the office door and asked if she could borrow the phone as she needed to speak to me. Obviously, the nurse had to dial the number but that was the last time I ever got a call from Mum and it is another cherished memory.

After four months in hospital, we were told that Mum was as good as she was going to get and we needed to agree the next steps. One option was for Mum to return home, although I think we knew in our hearts that we wouldn't be able to cope. However, a home visit was arranged with a member of staff from the hospital. I remember when we got back to the house the nurse asked Mum if she recognized where she was and she said, "No not really," which I found incredibly sad.

The visit didn't go well; Mum stumbled down a couple of stairs, quickly became agitated and started asking to go home. So with a heavy heart we all agreed that Mum needed to go into a care home.

20. Our story: Choosing a care home

Finding a suitable care home was made all the more stressful by the fact that the hospital staff and social services couldn't agree on the type of home needed.

We were given a list of care homes (with dementia care) and a list of nursing homes in the Scarborough region. Social services told us to concentrate on the nursing home list but then the hospital staff told us that a nursing home environment would be too restrictive for Mum and that she would be better in a care home setting.

What everyone agreed was that ideally, Mum needed somewhere with no stairs, which were a fall risk, and lots of room to 'pace' as Mum spent much of her time walking.

So we spent a few days going around all the homes on the list which was a truly soul-destroying exercise. As advised, we just turned up without notice, as you are more likely to get a true impression. There were a couple of homes that wouldn't let us look around when we arrived as they were too busy, so they were struck off the list. Then there was one home where I swear to this day that it was a resident who answered the door and told us to come back later!

Most of the homes we looked at were converted Victorian, three-storey houses, where the residents spent most of their time in one room, which would have driven Mum absolutely bonkers.

When we had just about exhausted the list we came across a care home in Scarborough, which was over two floors. However, the dementia unit was a secured area on the second floor which meant that Mum wouldn't have access to any stairs. It had many corridors for the residents to walk about and it had 24-hour access to the bedrooms.

A meeting was arranged with both hospital staff and social services to report back on our progress on finding a suitable home and to get an update on Mum. I remember we were sat in reception at Cross Lane updating the lady from social services that we had found a home which we thought would be ideal for Mum. You can imagine how unimpressed we were when she said, "That home will not be able to cater for your Mum's needs, she can't go there." Erm…excuse me for being pedantic but if it's not suitable for her, why was it on a list you gave us to look around?

I have to say that the meeting was a bit of a disaster. The hospital staff insisted that Mum attend the meeting, and I can appreciate that where possible, people with dementia should be involved in all aspects of their care. But as the meeting was primarily to discuss which care home was best for Mum (as a care home was the only feasible option) and Mum was adamant she wasn't going into a care home, it was never going to end well. It didn't help that Mum had a urine infection and was more confused, agitated and uncoordinated than usual and she got very upset right from the start. In the end, I had to take Mum out of the meeting and console her as she sobbed her heart out and told me that she would never forgive us for our treachery – that is the actual word she used and it was like a dagger through the heart.

Social services were adamant that the home we had picked wouldn't be able to cope with Mum and seemed to be pushing us to a particular home they had in mind, which we had looked around and dismissed. We were equally adamant that the only home we were happy with was the one they were saying was unsuitable.

So just when it looked like we had run out of options, and we were beginning to slightly panic, another option was proposed. Now granted it was near Malton, which is a 23-mile drive from Filey, but by this stage we would have considered anything. As it turned out Rivermead care home fit the bill perfectly. A specialised 'people centred care' dementia unit, on one floor with a secure central garden area, and plenty of room to roam.

A meeting was arranged with the head nurse for an assessment as to whether they felt they could cater for Mum's needs. We were keen to stress that we wanted to wait until Mum's infection had cleared up to give her the best possible chance of been accepted. I was there the day the assessment was done and I had a chat with the nurse from Cross Lane and the nurse from Rivermead. The nurse from Cross Lane, bless her, was trying to paint Mum in the best possible light, and thankfully Mum was accepted.

The day Mum left hospital and moved to Rivermead is another day that I will never forget. It was the 18th December 2013. It was obvious to Mum that something was happening as we packed her bags and waited for her to be signed off, but she didn't know what. Mum was quite anxious, as you would expect, but she was trying her best to stay positive. I can't remember what we told her but when we came to leave one of the nurses said, "All the best Chris, hope you settle well."

Mum replied, "Don't worry I will definitely be back later." I had to chuckle, she had spent the last 4 months trying to escape the place and now she was adamant she was coming back. Better the devil you know I suppose!

21. Our story: Rivermead care home

Mum was on the Memory Care unit at Rivermead, a specialised 'person centred care' dementia unit. Person centred care involves tailoring a person's care to their interests, abilities, history and personality. This helps them to take part in the things they enjoy and can also help carers to engage in reminiscence therapy (see chapter 22) both of which are effective ways of preventing and managing behavioural and psychological symptoms of dementia.

To our utter amazement, Mum seemed to settle really well into the care home and to some degree we got our old Mum back – one who wasn't always highly agitated and distressed. It was a really good environment for Mum because there was plenty of space to wander around, with a secure garden area. They also had an open bedroom door policy (many of the homes we looked around didn't) so Mum could have a nap if she was feeling tired – although not always in her own bed! This was something I personally felt quite passionate about. I don't know how you are supposed to call somewhere home if you can't even go into your own bedroom. It was also somewhere we could go and have some privacy when I visited, although for some reason everyone seemed to congregate in Mum's room so we didn't actually get much privacy.

I think one of the other main reasons that Mum seemed to settle, was because for the first time in a long time she was left alone and didn't have someone constantly checking up on her. The last year or so that she was at home, she couldn't really be left alone for longer than half an hour or so, and even then if she was sitting in the upstairs lounge and you heard her move, you had to go check she was ok because the stairs and furniture in the house were a trip/fall hazard. Then at Cross Lane, there was always a member of staff in the communal area so Mum never really got any peace. Whereas in Rivermead she could wander around and there were a number of rooms where she could just go and sit and enjoy a bit of peace and quiet.

Another factor I believe is that the layout of Rivermead largely mirrored a school and Mum would often talk as though she was at work. You would sometimes find her wandering around the communal dining room trying to get everyone to behave. I remember once when I arrived I could hear Mum saying, "The only voice I should be hearing is mine." Mum used to get very frustrated because nobody took a blind bit of notice!

Finally, because Mum was in a specialised dementia unit, all the other residents also had varying degrees of dementia, and while not everyone got on, largely they did. So there wasn't the underlying tension that there was at Cross Lane. In addition, because all the visitors had a loved one with dementia, if they spoke to Mum it was usually with a kindness and respect that you don't always get from people who have no experience of dementia.

Although she seemed relatively content, when Mum first arrived in the home she caused chaos and we were genuinely concerned that they wouldn't be able to cope. As I've mentioned they have an open bedroom door policy and Mum would wander into a bedroom, pick something up, get distracted and take it into the next bedroom, resulting in everyone's belongings been scattered to the four winds. She would also attempt to assist bedridden patients by either helping them out of bed or tucking them in, resulting in a risk of suffocation as she pulled the covers over people's heads. Fortunately, the home was very good at adapting, labelling everyone possessions and placing pressure mats in the doorways of all bedridden patients.

It was only after Mum went into Rivermead that I started to learn a little bit more about dementia with Lewy bodies – before then simply getting through the day was challenge enough. Although I had learnt the basics about the disease before, suddenly all the symptoms and behaviours that Mum had experienced from early on in her illness made sense. Understanding the disease made it seem less daunting somehow and it allowed me to relax more around Mum, which in turn reduced her anxiety around me. The fact that she had settled into a care home (something we thought would never happen) also helped to reduce the overwhelming burden of responsibility I had felt and meant that we could enjoy the time we spent together.

So we all settled into a routine. I would visit Mum a couple of times a week and stay most of the day. In the early days, I would arrive, we would go out for a walk and a coffee in a café, and then it would be back for lunch. After lunch, we would have a wander around the garden or just sit and have a chat. Those were happy days and are memories that I will always cherish.

Mum had always had a dry sense of humour and throughout her illness, she would amuse us all with her sharp wit. I remember one day my sister and I were visiting and laughing about something when Mum stopped laughing and said in a very serious tone, "Stop making me laugh in a hysterical way because I will wee." I don't think I stopped laughing for the rest of the day.

Mum was at Rivermead for just under 3 years and for a couple of years we would go out at least once a week but as Mum's illness progressed into the 3rd year, we stopped. One of the main problems was that Mum struggled to get in and out of the car but she would also get very tired, very quickly and couldn't walk very far. Another issue was toileting as she would suddenly need to go and it was a struggle to make it in time.

But although we no longer went out, we would still have a nice time. There was a reception area in Rivermead where you could go to sit and have a coffee and a cake. So we would often go for a little stroll around the garden (comfortable in the knowledge that if Mum became tired and stopped walking I could get help and a wheelchair to take her back) and then sit and have a coffee.

We would then go for lunch and while relatives of residents didn't get lunch (unless you paid for it) Mum would often 'blag' me some by saying, "Are you not having any?" and then insist on sharing her lunch with me. As a result, the staff would often load Mum's plate up with enough for both of us – good ploy Mum!

While visiting Mum I got to know the other residents who all had their own unique personalities and habits. In the third year of Mums stay a new resident, called June, came to live at Rivermead. June and Mum became good friends and they would wander around arm in arm for hours on end. June was there as Mum's health deteriorated and she would bring Mum apples from a tree in the garden and leave them on Mum's bed. Actually, she would throw them from the door and could have done some real damage but the thought was there.

There was another resident at Rivermead who had almost lost the ability to communicate but did have three words in her vocabulary, her name – Dot, Bugger and Off. Most of the conversations I had with her went as follows:

Me - "Morning."
Dot - "Bugger off."
Me - "Nice day."
Dot - "Bugger off."
Me - "What's your name?"
Dot - "Dot."
Me - "See you later then Dot."

Dot - "Bugger off."

Although not much of a conversationalist, Dot was good fun and she loved to be pushed around at great speed in her wheelchair, whooping with delight and shouting, "Bugger off."

There was another lady who was like a little 'Mini the Minx' (the comic book character) who would wander around looking for mischief. One day I saw her heading for a pile of plates with a grin on her face and before I could stop her she had tipped the whole pile on the floor. Shortly after that, she had a member of staff assigned to her at all times as she was such a little terror.

One of the downsides of getting to know the other residents was when they died. It was always upsetting to hear and you would miss them. It was also a reminder that dementia is a progressive disease (most of them anyway) and that you were slowly running out of time.

So while Rivermead wasn't perfect, they were often short-staffed and there were a couple of staff members who could be a little heavy-handed when helping Mum (not in an abusive way), on the whole, we couldn't really have hoped for a better place for Mum to spend her final years. In the main, the staff were great with Mum and I know that many of them grew very fond of her. I don't honestly know how I would have coped if Mum had ended up somewhere we weren't comfortable with and the worry that would have entailed.

So after 3 relatively happy and calm years, it was at Rivermead that Mum embarked on her final journey and finally passed away.

22. Dementia: Time-shift & reminiscence therapy

In some types of dementia, particularly Alzheimer's disease, the first part of the brain to be affected is the hippocampus, which plays a role in the formation of new memories. Although the hippocampus is required to retrieve newer memories, it isn't relied on so heavily to retrieve memories from longer ago. The amygdala, responsible for emotional memories, is also less affected in the earlier stages. This means that someone with Alzheimer's will struggle to remember what happened earlier that day but will be able to remember things that happened in their childhood and will be able to remember the emotional aspects of certain memories.

Note: Although short term memory problems may not be evident in the early stages of dementia with Lewy bodies, short term memory does become affected as the disease progresses.

When a person's short term memory is affected, they are more likely to interpret things in the present, based on memories of the past, as they are the memories that are most vivid. This is known as 'time-shift' and can result in them living in a different reality to yours. For example, Mum often believed she was of working age and would talk and act as though she was at school.

As the disease progresses further, they are more likely to regress back to their teenage years and early adulthood, as these memories often remain most vivid until the more advanced stages of dementia. This is known as the reminiscence bump (possibly due to the fact that a person's ability to remember new information peaks in our 20's).

As Mum's illness progressed she seemed to regress further back to the time when her parents were alive and she would often ask after her Dad. Handling questions like, "Have you seen my Dad?" when he has been dead for 30 years is a difficult one and is one reason why 'therapeutic lying' is commonplace in dementia care (see chapter 26).

Reminiscence therapy is an effective way to help positively engage with people who have 'time-shifted' and can help to manage some of the changes in behaviour that often occur in people living with dementia.

Reminiscence therapy is defined by the American Psychological Association (APA) as *the use of life histories – written, oral, or both – to improve psychological well-being* and is often used with older people.

How does it work?
Reminiscence therapy can be done with a professional, friend or relative, either in groups or on a one to one basis. It can be done with prompts, such as music, objects or photos. The prompts can be general, designed to trigger memories such as a piece of music from the 60s or specific to the person concerned, such as a photo of their wedding day.

In essence reminiscence therapy is simply acknowledging that someone has 'time-shifted' and is effectively living in the past. Past memories are the only ones that remain. So rather than constantly correcting them or engaging in conversations relating to things they know nothing about – because they occurred after the brain was damaged – you find things to talk about that they can remember, where they can contribute.

What are the benefits to the person living with dementia?

- ✓ Allows them to engage in conversation and recount happy memories.
- ✓ Reduces boredom.
- ✓ Improves mood.
- ✓ Increases confidence.
- ✓ Reminds them of their identity.
- ✓ Promotes a greater feeling of self-worth.

Note: Reminiscence therapy is less effective in the very advanced stages of dementia as the part of the brain which deals with longer term memories also becomes affected. I have also read that it is less effective for people living with frontotemporal dementia, possibly because memory loss isn't the primary symptom.

Mum & time-shift
I always tried to join Mum in her reality. I tried to talk about things in the past or kept the conversation very general.

Having said that, I do remember one conversation

where I managed to upset Mum as I didn't acknowledge she had time-shifted.

Mum - "Sorry what's your name again?"
Me - "Emma, I'm your eldest daughter."
Mum - "How old are you?"
Me - "45."
Mum - "Right, well how old am I?"
Me - "72."
Mum - "72, 72 that can't be right!"

A moments silence occurred while I tried to think of a suitable reply when Mum suddenly said with a hint of emotion, "Bloody Hell, how did that happen!"

I quickly changed the subject and avoided talking about age ever again. Bless!

23. Dementia: Communication

Aphasia is a condition that leads to either a partial or total loss of the ability to comprehend and formulate language, verbally or using written word. Aphasia can affect a person's ability to find the right words, to understand what others are saying, to recognize the names of objects, and can also affect reading and writing. Aphasia is caused by a brain injury or disease (such as dementia).

I always knew that dementia will gradually affect the way a person communicates. Their ability to present rational ideas and to reason clearly will change. I knew that a person with dementia may have trouble finding the right word, they may repeat words and phrases, or may become 'stuck' mid-sentence.

But what I didn't necessarily appreciate is that they may continue to talk, but without any meaning. Mum used to talk for hours but as her illness progressed most of what she said stopped making any sense. She would put 'jumbled up' words together to make incomprehensible sentences.

It always struck me though that what she was saying made sense to her because occasionally she would say something and then ask, "What do you think?" Difficult to answer as I didn't have a clue what she had just said and if my response wasn't the one she was obviously looking for she would get upset.

The technique I learnt to apply in those situations was to say, "Erm, I'm not sure, what do you think?" she would then tell me what she thought and I would still be none the wiser!

It isn't easy communicating with someone who is making no sense and I came across a lot of people who simply dismissed Mum as soon as she started talking to them, as they didn't know how to respond. When this happened Mum would get very embarrassed, upset and would become very quiet. It would really knock her confidence and I think it is one of the easiest ways to rob someone with dementia of their dignity.

Knowing the devastating impact this had on Mum is the reason why I am including this chapter. I always found that the occasional 'yes, that's right' or something equally as vague would allow the conversation to continue. And however the conversation was going, if she asked me a question, I would always supply the best answer I could. In other words, we engaged in a conversation, even if her half and my half of the conversation bore no relation to each other.

As Mum's illness progressed she started to use words that didn't exist. So rather than just jumbling up actual words to make a sentence that made no sense, it was as though she was jumbling up the letters to make words that made no sense. It still didn't stop her from talking though; it just made it more difficult to realize when she was expecting a response.

Below are some tips on improving communication but my main advice is just 'go with the flow,' don't be embarrassed and respond as though you have understood, even when you haven't.

Tips for successful communication

- ✓ Where possible, approach the person with dementia from the front.
- ✓ Minimize other distractions such as the television, radio or other people's conversation.
- ✓ Maintain eye contact. If the person is sitting, drop down to their eye level. Standing over someone can be intimidating.
- ✓ Speak clearly and calmly.
- ✓ Make sentences short and simple.
- ✓ Try to avoid questions that require complicated answers.
- ✓ Don't repeat questions that might embarrass them like 'Don't you remember?'
- ✓ Ask one question at a time, too many choices can be confusing and frustrating.
- ✓ Processing information will take the person longer than it used to, so be patient. Don't hurry them as they may feel under pressure.
- ✓ Be aware of nonverbal communication; look for the feelings behind the words.

When you don't understand what someone is communicating

- ✓ Listen actively and carefully.
- ✓ Focus on a word or phrase that does make sense.

- ✓ Respond to the emotional tone of the sentence, not the words.
- ✓ Stay calm and be patient.
- ✓ Ask family members about possible meaning for words, names and phrases.
- ✓ Respond as though you understand.
- ✓ If necessary try a hug and change the subject.
- ✓ Simply reply ok or fab.

Things not to do

- ✓ Don't argue.
- ✓ Don't order the person around.
- ✓ Don't tell the person what they can and cannot do.
- ✓ Don't be condescending.
- ✓ Don't talk about people in front of them.
- ✓ Do not talk over or through a person as if they are not there.
- ✓ Avoid whispering as it creates suspicion.
- ✓ Don't patronize the person or ridicule what they say.

24. Our story: Later stages

Once Mum settled into Rivermead, her level of anxiety and agitation reduced dramatically. However, as her dementia progressed, new challenges and behaviours started to emerge.

Simple everyday tasks such as dressing, toileting, eating and even sitting down in a chair became more difficult. Once Mum got to the advanced stages, almost everything became a monumental, time-consuming effort.

From very early on in her illness Mum had struggled to choose what to eat if she was presented with more than one option. In the early/mid stages of the disease, once the food arrived she would manage to eat it herself, including cutting up her food and using a knife and folk. As the disease progressed she firstly needed help cutting up the food, then switched to using a spoon when a knife and fork became too difficult. She then started struggling with a spoon and tended to use her fingers and eventually needed spoon-feeding.

Toileting became ridiculously difficult. Although she was fine whilst she was at home, when she went into Cross Lane and at Rivermead, she needed help finding the toilet but then could manage herself. She then started to struggle a bit and needed prompting on the different stages – of which there are more than you would think! Then in the later stages, she needed help with every stage but she used to get incredibly embarrassed, which would often result in quite aggressive behaviour.

Even sitting down in a chair became very difficult for Mum. Perhaps as a result of the problems with spatial awareness (see chapter 36), Mum would hold the arm of the chair, before she would lower herself onto it. But she would often misjudge and miss the chair, ending up on the floor. I came up with a technique where I would use my legs to help manoeuvre her into the correct position if it looked like she was going to miss. I also learnt that if a chair was quite low with no arms there would be no chance she would even attempt to sit down – which I found out to my cost in a café one day!

As the disease progressed, Mum's behaviour became more bizarre, but to be fair to her there was always a bit of logic behind her actions. If we decided to go for a walk for example, and went to her room for a coat, she would often pull a jumper out of her wardrobe and start trying to put it on her head. She obviously wanted a hat but got a bit muddled.

Often when we would go for a coffee and a cake, she would unwrap the cake and drop it straight in her coffee. One day I casually enquired what she was doing when she replied, "Warming it up." Fair enough, can't fault the logic!

Another strange habit Mum had was stuffing a load of clothes down the toilet and when I asked her about it she would always reply, "I was just putting a wash on."

Mum also became more unaware of the normal boundaries of social etiquette. She had a habit of commenting (loudly) about the size of overweight people. She wasn't being nasty or malicious, she was just being truthful, saying things other people would only think (but not say out loud). Once I tried to explain that it wasn't the 'done thing' but she genuinely couldn't understand what the problem was. It got to the point where if I saw an overweight person approaching I would change direction to avoid hurting anyone's feelings.

Strangely though, as Mum's illness progressed and there was a general decline in her cognition and her behaviour became more bizarre, she still never ceased to amaze me. For example, she could still recite her old telephone number and date of birth, even when she couldn't remember my name. And long after her ability to communicate effectively was gone i.e. when she had started jumbling up words to make sentences, she could still read out loud a sign or a newspaper headline.

As dementia progresses communication and every aspect of daily living becomes more difficult and time-consuming. Behaviours can seem strange and illogical. Personally though, I found the later stages easier and while I accept that it is largely down to the fact that Mum was in a care home and was no longer highly agitated, it was partly because I understood the disease better and I learnt to 'enter into her reality.'

The other thing I learnt is to never be surprised by a person with dementia, however advanced their disease. Never underestimate their abilities or their capacity for love and laughter. Some of my most cherished memories are from when Mum was in the more advanced stages of the disease.

25. Lewy who: Stages of Lewy body dementia

Although the rate of progression varies from person to person, dementia is generally described as going through 3 stages – mild or early, moderate or mid and severe or late.

For more meaningful terms between professionals, caregivers and patients, a more detailed process in 7 stages, has been described for Alzheimer's disease.

One question many people have is what are the stages of Lewy body dementia? Unfortunately throughout my research, I have never come across a similar definitive breakdown of the stages of dementia with Lewy bodies. So below is a breakdown of how Mum's illness progressed.

Precursor to dementia with Lewy bodies

Mum suffered from REM sleep behaviour disorder and a loss of sense of smell, years before the first noticeable symptoms of dementia with Lewy bodies appeared and they are thought to be possible precursor symptoms of Lewy body dementia.

✓ REM sleep behaviour disorder (physically acting out vivid dreams with vocal sounds and sudden arm and leg movement) may be one of the first symptoms of Parkinson's disease or a Lewy body dementia. Doctors have recognized that patients may have REM sleep behaviour disorder years before other symptoms of

Parkinson's or a Lewy body dementia appear (see chapter 38).

✓ Newcastle University carried out a study to identify symptoms closely associated with Lewy body dementia, before the onset of dementia, and a loss of sense of smell was also one of the earliest symptoms reported by participants. However as a loss of smell is common in healthy older adults and people with Alzheimer's disease, it is not specific enough to suggest it is a precursor symptom of Lewy body dementia – although it was for Mum.

Early Stages

The symptoms that Mum experienced from very early in her illness included:

✓ Restlessness.
✓ Changes in mood becoming depressed, anxious and agitated.
✓ Loss of initiative, interests.
✓ Fluctuating cognition.
✓ Ability to perform daily tasks affected such as making tea/coffee.
✓ Hallucinations.
✓ Delusions.
✓ Problems with spatial awareness i.e. problems walking up/down stairs.
✓ Some movement difficulties including shuffling walk when tired and poor coordination.
✓ Dizziness on standing.
✓ Increased daytime sleep: two-plus hours.

✓ Chronic runny nose, we couldn't leave the house without a box of tissues!

Middle Stages

As Mum's illness progressed she became less anxious (possibly due to medication) but along with the symptoms listed above she also started to experience the following:

✓ Symptoms developed that more strongly resemble Parkinson's including slight hand tremor and occasional muscle jerk.
✓ More frequent falls.
✓ Difficulty with speech and finding words (aphasia). Although Mum talked a lot, as the disease progressed much of what she said stopped making sense.
✓ Impaired ability to swallow.
✓ Declining cognition.
✓ Handwriting affected (often smaller or less legible).
✓ Inability to tell time or comprehend time passing.
✓ Started to struggle to recognize family members.

Later Stages

During the last year or so of her life, Mum moved to what I would class as the later stages of the disease and became increasingly frail and confused – although she still continued to have moments of clarity right until the end of her life. Additional symptoms included:

✓ Extreme muscle rigidity and sensitivity to touch.

- ✓ Struggled to walk far, becoming tired very quickly.
- ✓ Very unsteady on feet.
- ✓ Frequent falls.
- ✓ Became susceptible to infections (urinary and chest).
- ✓ Greater difficulty swallowing.
- ✓ Decline in language – started to use words that made no sense.
- ✓ Incontinent of bladder and occasionally bowel.
- ✓ Increased daytime sleeping.
- ✓ Needed assistance with all aspects of daily living.

Throughout her illness, there was a gradual decline in Mum's physical strength and cognition, although her cognition did continue to fluctuate so you did get good days where she seemed quite 'with it' even in the very late stages. However, in the much later stages (final year) frequent falls and infections did mean that the decline was more rapid.

26. Dementia: Therapeutic lies

The term 'therapeutic lie' is a false statement or deception with the best interest of the patient at heart. Therapeutic lying is commonplace in caring for people with dementia and it is a dilemma that many caregivers and healthcare professionals struggle with.

- ✓ Some people think that telling a therapeutic lie is the right thing to do. They feel that it is easier, kinder and avoids upset which can lead to changes in behaviour.
- ✓ Some people think that it is the wrong thing to do, that it is deceitful and disrespectful and cannot be justified.
- ✓ Finally there are those who think it is better to try and distract the person with dementia, or perhaps slightly bend the truth, rather than tell an outright lie.

Some caregiver may also worry that the trust that they have with the person living with dementia may be broken if they are 'caught out' by lying.

I personally had no problem with telling therapeutic lies to Mum. As mentioned before, Mum often used to ask, "Have you seen my Dad?" So rather than tell her that he had been dead for 30 years, I used to lie and tell her he had just nipped to the shops. She was always satisfied with this response and I know that if I told her he was dead she would have been upset and distressed.

If I knew I only had to tell her he had died once, and that she would remember, I would have considered being truthful. But she asked me the same question every week and I personally could not see any benefit in causing undue upset, time and time again. I certainly didn't feel as though I was in any way being disrespectful.

In fact, I used to do anything in my power to keep Mum happy and content. I used to basically agree with everything she said and seeing as though I very rarely had any idea what she was saying, technically I wasn't lying!

Although I personally had no problem with lying to Mum (although I preferred to think of it as entering her reality, the one where her Dad was still alive), I knew Mum, knew what would upset her and what calmed her. I can however, appreciate it may be more difficult to use therapeutic lies with someone you don't know so well, when you're not so sure of the reaction you may get.

27. Our story: The final journey

We can pinpoint the beginning of the end of Mum's journey to the 23rd June 2016. I was at home when I received a call from the care home to say that Mum's condition had deteriorated badly. I remember saying, "Do we need to be there?"

The nurse replied, "If it was my Mum, I would want to be here."

So we all rushed over and Mum seemed to be having some sort of fit. She had lost the ability to speak, couldn't focus, was constantly twitching and seemed to be in a certain amount of distress. They gave her a sedative and she went to sleep. The following day she seemed calmer but still couldn't speak or focus. The doctor came and advised us, that in his opinion she had had some sort of brain incident, probably a stroke, but without any investigation he couldn't be sure.

We were then asked whether Mum should:

a) Be admitted to hospital for a brain scan to establish what had happened (which would be highly distressing), even though it is likely that little could be done as no surgeon would agree to operate on someone with such advanced dementia.

b) Leave her in the home, which was familiar to her, where she could be kept comfortable and pain-free. Even though, while she may rally for a while, the likelihood is that she would die.

Rightly or wrongly we chose option b) and fully expected the worse. By this stage, Mum couldn't swallow properly and couldn't focus or speak. She certainly couldn't get out of bed. Imagine our surprise when each day she started to improve and within a week she was eating solid food, speech and focus back to normal and she was even walking albeit a bit wobbly.

But it wasn't to be and over the next three months, Mum suffered one thing after another. She never really regained her mobility, although that didn't stop her from trying to walk, and as a result she had repeated falls and on one occasion was hospitalized as a result. She always seemed to have a urine infection and she also suffered a chest infection. As a result, there was a dramatic decline in her dementia symptoms. In addition, there were a couple more brain incidents, similar but less severe, than the one that marked the beginning of the end.

Approximately a month before Mum died we received a call to say that Mum had been taken to hospital with a swollen stomach. Steve and I rushed to the hospital and Mum's stomach was absolutely huge, she looked like she was 9 months pregnant. After an initial examination, it was discovered that Mum's bowel was full but at that stage, they didn't know the cause. They administered an enema, which seemed to work and Mum was admitted overnight so they could continue giving her regular enemas to clear her bowel.

The following day I was there when the consultant visited and we had the familiar conversation – we could do some tests to find out the cause of the blockage, it may be a number of things including a cancerous tumour, but it would be quite invasive and whatever the cause it's unlikely that surgery would be performed. So Mum was released from hospital on the proviso that she would be given regular enemas to keep her bowels clear. Mum took the hospital visit completely in her stride, which was an indication of just how poorly she was, as usually, she would have been hysterical given the treatment she had to endure.

There is a caravan site down the road from Rivermead and for the final three months of Mum's life, we took our caravan there often. In the final month of Mum's life we practically moved in and I feel very blessed that I got to spend so much time with her, time I knew I would never get back.

As Mum became weaker and weaker, she still always recognized me as someone she knew and loved and I hold on tightly to that fact. One day, a week or so before she died, she was in bed barely able to move. I lay next to her and put my head on her shoulder when suddenly I felt her gently kiss the top of my head. I remember feeling completely overwhelmed with love and emotion as I sobbed into her shoulder.

By now Mum had become almost entirely immobile and spent much of her time sleeping. Over the next few weeks, she became weaker and weaker and started eating less and less. Eventually, she lost the ability to swallow and stopped eating altogether. We then knew the inevitable was within sight.

28. Dementia: Dysphagia

A common symptom as dementia progresses is difficulty in swallowing – known as dysphagia. Although dysphagia can be present in different types of dementia, it is much more common in dementia with Lewy bodies than in Alzheimer's disease.

Dysphagia can increase the risk of aspiration (food going down the wrong way into the lungs), choking, poor nutrition and a reduced quality of life.

Although this didn't become a problem for Mum until the much later stages, you could argue that it is what ultimately caused her death, as she simply lost the ability to swallow and therefore could no longer eat or drink anything.

I had always been happy to help Mum during mealtimes, firstly helping her choose food which I knew she would enjoy the most. I also used to make sure Mum wasn't given anything that was too chewy, partly because she had lost most of her teeth due to her aversion to dentists. I would then cut up her food and help to get it onto her fork or spoon. Then when Mum became unable to use a knife/fork/spoon, I would happily feed her.

In the months leading up to Mum's death, swallowing started to become more and more of a problem and she would simply stop chewing halfway through a mouthful and 'pocket' the food in her cheeks. I found that massaging the back of her neck and rubbing her cheeks prompted her to chew and then rubbing the front of her neck seemed to help her swallow. Eventually Mum had to go onto pureed food and thickened liquid as she was simply unable to chew food sufficiently and would start to choke on un-thickened liquids.

It was around this time that I became less confident in helping Mum at mealtimes, worried that she would start choking. I was never sure that the food had actually gone down as there was no longer a 'clear swallow,' so would be really reluctant to give her the next spoonful.

In the last month or so of Mum's life, I stopped feeding her altogether, as I just couldn't cope with the gurgling sound she tended to make, thinking she was choking. I wish now that I had spent a bit more time learning how to recognize what was safe, as I would have been able to devote more time than the staff could, to feeding Mum small amounts of food.

Below is a summary of some of the techniques that can be used to help with dysphagia:

- ✓ Feed slowly, allowing time to chew.
- ✓ Remind to swallow.
- ✓ Try offering an empty cup or spoon to prompt a swallow.
- ✓ Offer fluids frequently.
- ✓ Check for pocketed food or liquid in cheeks.
- ✓ Place food on the strong side of the mouth.
- ✓ Encourage highly flavoured food and drinks, as these provide more stimulation to the brain to prompt a swallow response.

- ✓ Offer soft or pureed food/thickened liquids.
- ✓ Make sure they're sitting upright and are as calm and comfortable as possible before you begin.
- ✓ Keep the eating area free from distractions.

29. Our story: The end

At the point when Mum became gravely ill, I knew quite a lot about dementia with Lewy bodies but I had never researched what to expect at end of life. I have since learnt that the signs that death may be very close include:

- ✓ Drifting into unconsciousness.
- ✓ Inability to swallow.
- ✓ Irregular 'stop/start' breathing.
- ✓ Cold hands and feet.
- ✓ Agitation or restlessness.

I have also learnt that once someone has lost the ability to swallow then oral care is administered to try and keep the person as comfortable as possible. Mum was given oral swabs (a small sponge on a stick which is dipped in liquid and used to moisten and refresh the mouth), below are some tips on best practice.

Oral Care at end of life

- ✓ Mouth care should be done two hourly or more frequently if required to keep the mouth moist.
- ✓ Use any fluids familiar to the person to swab the mouth such as tea or coffee, fruit juice or even alcohol if they used to enjoy a drink. It is the act of moistening the mouth and not the fluid you use that is important.
- ✓ Consider using ice cream or yoghurt if it isn't a choking risk.

- ✓ Avoid anything that is too hot, to avoid burning or too cold which can be a shock.
- ✓ Saliva spray can also be used to moisten the mouth.
- ✓ Only use gentle pressure with swabs or a toothbrush.
- ✓ Take care not to put a toothbrush or swab near the back of the mouth or it may cause gagging.
- ✓ Teeth can also be gently cleaned with water and a soft toothbrush, which will help keep the mouth fresh.
- ✓ Keep an eye out for ulcers or sores and treat accordingly.
- ✓ Apply lip balm which helps to keep the person comfortable.

I have to say that I wish I had done some research earlier, as I was totally unprepared for the last few days of Mum's life. Mum did become totally unresponsive, unable to move or speak and often seemed to be asleep. She did lose the ability to swallow and became very dehydrated as a result. Her breathing was laboured, and as a result of a lack of oxygen, her feet and hands did become cold and then along with her lips and ears started to turn blue. Thankfully, for the majority of the time, Mum didn't appear to be in pain or distress and didn't seem agitated or restless, although there were a couple of times when she did become agitated. The first time simply repositioning her in bed seemed to do the trick but the second time she was given an injection (I think it was a mild sedative).

My sister and I spent the final weekend with Mum who finally died on Monday 26th September 2016. The day my world changed forever.

At the beginning of the weekend, Mum's breathing became more laboured and she seemed to have a lot of fluid/mucus in her throat, making a horrible rasping sound when she breathed. The nurse tried to 'suction' the mucus away to clear her chest and she was also given something that dries up secretions, which seemed to work.

By this point, Mum was totally dehydrated and even giving oral care swabs was difficult because Mum would suck on it and then start choking. So it had to be done with a fairly dry swab and even then she kept clamping her mouth shut and refusing to open it. I think it was her way of saying, will you stop sticking things in my mouth and just get me a Gin & Tonic!

I totally accept that someone with dementia, at the end of life, starts refusing food and drink (often because they lose the ability to swallow) and become dehydrated. I don't believe in Mums case that we should have initiated intravenous fluids, to prolong life; I totally accept that she was following a natural progression to death.

However, I don't think we did enough to keep Mum comfortable. The oral mouth swabs were not given every two hours. I found it really hard to give Mum the swabs, because not only did she suck on them and start choking but she also tried to bite the sponge part off –

probably because she was so desperate for some hydration. Although I wasn't comfortable administering the swabs, had I known I would have tried using a toothbrush instead, as I would have been more comfortable that she wouldn't have managed to bite the end off. In addition, I would have used Gin & Tonic to swab her mouth, as I believe it would have been more refreshing than water.

On reflection, I also remember that there was mention of a saliva spray that can be used, which we didn't. I was so distraught at the time that I didn't retain that information; it wasn't mentioned again and was never used.

Mum's breathing continued to become more shallow and laboured, which I know is common with dementia patients, and although I have read it isn't distressing for them, I don't know how we can know that.

She actually died at 16.44 pm although she first stopped breathing an hour earlier than that and then started again. For the next hour, she would stop breathing and then start again, gasping for breath. Although again I have been told that this is common in dementia patients, it was beyond horrific and that last hour, in particular, will haunt my dreams forever. To my mind, to have someone who is so desperate to get breath into their lungs, their jaw cracks, can only be described as barbaric and to be told that its 'the norm' seems unacceptable.

However, I also accept that it wasn't appropriate to give

Mum any oxygen, artificially prolonging life. But once someone is literally gasping for breath, as she was for the last few hours of life, surely something could be done to help them slip away – as a cancer patient in extreme pain, would be given morphine.

Because Mum didn't appear to be in any distress, no medication was given. But just because she didn't appear to be in any distress, by this point she was fairly unresponsive so we will never know for sure. However, in my view gasping for breath and being totally dehydrated must be incredibly uncomfortable and frightening.

Throughout the final week or so of Mum's life, we kept being told that everything she went through was as you would expect. Well, it certainly wasn't what I was expecting and I feel that we should have been better prepared. Although nobody wants to hear in horrific detail, what their loved one is going to go through, if you are going to witness it anyway, surely it is better to be forewarned.

In hindsight, we should have had a meeting with a nurse and gone through what was likely to happen and what could be done to help alleviate the symptoms. We should have been told how often the oral swabs should be administered and agreed by whom. We should have been taught how to administer the saliva spray and agreed if we were comfortable doing it.

So I would like to say that Mum had a peaceful death but I don't think she did. I now realize we could have done more to help keep her more comfortable in terms of hydration. And whilst I know, under the current laws, we probably couldn't have done anything about Mum's breathing; I am now a firm believer of assisted dying. Given the choice, once Mum's breathing had become so shallow she had started to turn blue (the point at which it is fairly safe to say there is no coming back) I would have defiantly helped Mum to die, and saved her those last few difficult hours of her life.

Although the last few days of Mum's life were traumatic, there were some lighter moments. Many of the other residents used to regularly wander into Mum's room and although we could have locked the door to prevent it, we didn't feel it was appropriate – partly because they would resort to kicking the door, which unsettled Mum. Mum's friend June used to regularly check on whether she was any better and the day before Mum died she wandered in for about the fifth time and said simply, "Is she dead yet?" When we assured her that she wasn't June said, "Well that's good then," and wandered off.

During that final weekend, another resident wandered in, looked out of the window and asked for a 'leg up' as she wanted to go home. She started to get quite agitated as we were trying to explain that the window didn't open far enough, when she turned around towards us. I think she was about to tell us off (which she did often) when she looked at Mum and said, "I can see you've enough on, I'll find another way." Bless!

30. Our story: Timeline

The average life expectancy for people with dementia with Lewy bodies is 5 to 8 years after the onset of symptoms. Although Mum's journey fell into that range, some people have been known to live between 2 and 20 years with it, depending on their age and other medical conditions they may have.

Mum was a relatively young 67 years of age in 2009 when the first symptoms appeared. Although there is no doubt that there was a gradual decline in her cognitive functioning and physical strength, up until the first brain incident in June 2016, which marked the beginning of the end of her life, Mum was fairly well and we thought she would go on for years.

I believe one of the hardest things with dementia is not knowing how much time you have left. Knowing that the inevitable will happen, that they will forget your name, they will lose the ability to speak, they will die, but not knowing when each of these milestones will occur, leaves you in a state of limbo, unable to make any firm plans for life ahead.

Below is a rough timeline (as best as I can remember) of Mum's journey, one that fell into the average range of life expectancy.

Date	Milestone
June 2009	First remembered symptoms appear but barely noticeable at the time. There was just a general feeling that Mum was more vague and unorganised than usual.
June 2009 – October 2011	More noticeable symptoms seemed to appear suddenly and dramatically but unable to be more specific.
Circa End 2010 / Early 2011	Started process of trying to get a diagnosis with initial visit to the doctors.
October 2011	Very obvious symptoms evident including unable to remember details, repetitive questioning and general confusion (key date remembered due to repetitive questioning about a holiday).
March 2012	Received incorrect diagnosis of mixed Alzheimer's disease and vascular dementia.
Circa End 2012 / Early 2013	Received correct diagnosis of dementia with Lewy bodies.
August 2013	Mum was hospitalised due to dramatic decline in cognition and behaviour.
December 2013	Mum moved to Rivermead care home.
June 2016	Brain incident which resulted in short term loss of all movement, speech and ability to focus.
June 2016 / September 2016	Numerous infections, falls and illnesses resulting in a rapid decline in both physical and cognitive abilities.
September 2016	Mum died on the 26th September 2016. Cause of death recorded as Lewy body dementia.

31. Lewy who: The most challenging symptoms

I don't claim to be an expert in dementia and have very little experience of Alzheimer's disease or any other type of dementia. However, from what I have observed from other residents in the care home where Mum lived, and from what I have read and researched, I truly believe that dementia with Lewy bodies is the most challenging type of dementia to manage.

Dementia with Lewy bodies is unique because not only is cognition affected, which happens with other types of dementia, but movement and autonomic processes (key involuntary functions such as breathing, heart rate, digestive processes and body temperature) are also affected.

In addition, cognitive symptoms, such as hallucinations and problems with visual perception, appear early in the progression of the disease whereas with Alzheimer's, for example, the same symptoms do not appear until later.

Because these very challenging symptoms occur in the earlier stages of the disease, the loss of independence happens much sooner, which has a significant impact on both the person living with dementia and their caregivers.

Also, there are few approved drugs available for the treatment of dementia with Lewy bodies, there is only limited evidence about what treatments work and everyone responds differently. Another problem is that medication prescribed to improve cognition or hallucinations can make movement problems worse and vice/versa. People with dementia with Lewy bodies may also have a severe reaction to antipsychotic drugs, which are often used to treat hallucinations, a common feature of the disease (see chapter 16).

Finally, as well as coping with these challenging symptoms, there is a lack of knowledge both in the public and private sectors. This increases feelings of isolation and leads to a lack of trust in the medical establishment.

The Lewy Body Dementia Association conducted a survey which concluded that - Early and distinguishing characteristics of Lewy body dementias (LBD) are associated with higher levels of LBD caregiver subjective burden (how caregivers appraise the emotional, physical and social challenges they experience), over and above the effects of typical stressors found in other types of dementia. Key factors in LBD caregiver burden included behavioural problems, an impaired ability to perform activities of daily living, the LBD caregiver's sense of isolation, and challenges with the diagnostic experience.

I would say we experienced all the key factors mentioned above, in particular early behavioural problems caused by Mum's anxiety, her early loss of independence due to her inability to perform even the most basic tasks of daily living and challenges getting a diagnosis.

I believe that in order to be able to provide adequate care for someone with dementia with Lewy bodies, you have to understand the disease. I certainly wish I had understood some of the symptoms that occurred early in Mum's illness, and how to manage them, much sooner. I truly believe that it would have made the journey much easier for all of us as we could have reduced Mum's anxiety, increased her confidence and kept her at home for longer.

Therefore, the following few chapters cover the symptoms we found most challenging, how we dealt with them and what we learnt along the way.

32. Lewy who: Fluctuating cognition

Fluctuating cognition is a very difficult symptom to manage as it makes it very difficult to plan the level of care your loved one needs. They can change from someone who is capable of been left on their own to needing someone around to keep them safe, within the space of a few hours.

The fluctuations can last from minutes to hours to days and can be interspersed with periods of near-normal functioning. The severity, type and duration of symptoms can vary from a brief decline in the ability to perform daily tasks, to extreme confusion, disorganised speech or bizarre behaviour.

Mum's behaviour did fluctuate throughout the day. If the previous day had been particularly challenging, I would arrange to go and spend the following morning with Mum to give Steve a break, only to find Mum on great form. There were also times when I had cared for Mum in the morning, which had passed without incident, so I had left feeling comfortable that things were fine, only to receive a call a couple of hours later because Mum had become particularly distressed or had gone missing.

Mum's fluctuations could be quite extreme and she would go from near-normal functioning to becoming extremely confused and/or agitated throughout the day. I seem to recall that a 'nap' could precipitate the change, so she could be ok, fall asleep and then be 'all over the place' once she woke up.

Another challenge for caregivers is that fluctuating cognition can mislead other people's perception of the severity of the dementia symptoms. For example, if you get a visitor during a period of near-normal functioning, they potentially go away thinking things are fine and that no further support is needed.

I recall Mum always seemed to perform better when there were other people around, as though she put all her powers of concentration into staying more focussed to avoid becoming embarrassed. Although this was good for her, it is easy to become slightly resentful because believe me, when you are at the end of your tether, it can be very frustrating when those around you don't appreciate what you're going through.

Fluctuations also didn't help when we were dealing with her assigned consultant psychiatrist and community psychiatric nurse (CPN). I would put in an emergency call to the CPN, advising her that Mum was still highly agitated and asking for advice on what to do. She would arrange a home visit and Mum would often be absolutely fine when she arrived.

It wasn't only Mum's behaviour and general confusion that fluctuated throughout the day but also her ability to perform tasks. In June 2016 I bought a birthday card for Mum to sign for Kate. Below left is the first attempt at writing – To Kate, Love from Mum – not overly successful. Later in the day, Mum seemed less confused so we had another attempt, below right. As you can see there is a marked difference between the two, which were written only a couple of hours apart.

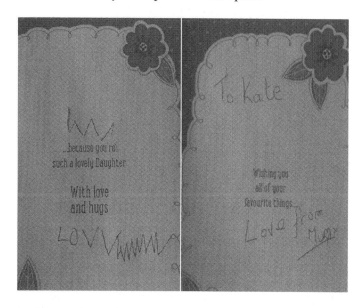

As Mum's behaviour started to deteriorate – and to overcome the fact that Mum always seemed fine when there was a healthcare professional about – we started keeping an hour by hour diary of how she was in terms of her general alertness, confusion and agitation levels. If Mum was particularly anxious I would also video her on my phone as evidence of just how agitated she could become. This really helped because we had an accurate hour by hour account of her fluctuations, rather than having to recall how she had been when trying to update our CPN.

It was this diary that eventually led to Mum been hospitalised when it became apparent that, although

Mum did have periods of relative normality, her behaviour had reached a point where she had potentially become a danger to herself and others.

33. Lewy who: Hallucinations

Visual hallucinations affect 2 out of 3 people with dementia with Lewy bodies. These hallucinations range from well-formed images of people (often children) or animals to more abstract visions such as shapes and colours.

From very early on in her illness, Mum experienced visual hallucinations and it was one of the things I found most upsetting and difficult to deal with.

The first time it happened I didn't appreciate Mum was hallucinating. I heard her talking but when I went into the room there was no one there. I just thought she was talking to herself, as I'm sure we all do from time to time. This was before we had a diagnosis of dementia with Lewy bodies and it never entered my mind that she was actually talking to someone who she could 'see.'

As it started to happen more and more, I would often find Mum stood up gesticulating and talking as though she was having a really animated conversation with someone and the name Mary seemed to crop up a lot – Mum did have a family member called Mary.

Although I would often find Mum talking to 'thin air' there were also common themes to her hallucinations. Firstly in a morning, she would often get very agitated as she needed to take the register and the 'kids' wouldn't get into line. It was obvious she was 'seeing' children and she would start chastising them for misbehaving. Mum was a teacher so that may have influenced why this particular hallucination was common for her.

The home Mum lived in was a three-story house, with the kitchen and dining room on the ground floor and the living room on the first floor. Mum was not only convinced that it wasn't her house but she was also convinced that there was a strange family living on the ground floor, which only strengthened her conviction that it wasn't her house.

In the early days, we used to spend hours trying to convince Mum that there was nobody there and I now realize that this was the wrong thing to do. The visual hallucinations that people with dementia with Lewy bodies see are as real to them as the world we see is to us. Trying to convince her otherwise simply led her to distrust us, increasing her anxiety, paranoia and delusions.

Later, once I understood more about hallucinations, whilst I didn't encourage them, I would generally just leave her be unless she started to get upset or agitated. If this happened I would then try and distract her onto something else and I found this to be the best approach.

I always got the impression that Mum's hallucination were just visual and not auditory because you would often find her repeating the same question over and over, obviously not getting any response from whoever she was conversing with. I once found Mum 'chatting away' to 'someone' and she was getting a bit agitated when she suddenly said to me, "Why won't they answer me?"

So I replied, "They seem a bit tired to me Mum, why don't we go and get a coffee, and try again later." She was happy with this response and we didn't need to try again later as the moment had passed.

Fortunately for us, Mum's hallucinations very rarely seemed to upset or distress her. In the early days, it was the fact that we used to try and convince her that there was nobody there that caused the upset. So while at first it can be very disconcerting and upsetting when your loved one is hallucinating, you have to remember that the part of the brain that controls vision is damaged and they are seeing something that is very real to them. Trying to convince them otherwise will often do more harm than good.

34. Lewy who: Multitasking and problem solving

People with Alzheimer's disease do not store information about what happens now, so are unable to remember the present. Whereas people with dementia with Lewy bodies, have more trouble retrieving information that has already been stored. In addition, people with dementia with Lewy bodies tend to lose their thinking skills sooner than a person with Alzheimer's. As a result, they quickly lose their ability to perform even the most basic tasks, particularly in the correct order, impacting early on their quality of life.

I once read that if you imagine that everyone has all the information about how to carry out each step of everyday tasks, stored in filing cabinets in their head. Well for people with dementia with Lewy bodies, it is like a bomb has gone off. Therefore rather than having everything neatly stored, step by step in their brain, they just have one single pile of information. So while all the information is still there, it is difficult to retrieve it and almost impossible to retrieve several steps in the right order.

From very early on in her illness, Mum struggled with some of the most basic everyday tasks. In fact, much of what Mum enjoyed doing before her illness, such as reading, cooking and gardening, she simply stopped doing altogether. So we didn't necessarily notice she was struggling with these tasks because she didn't even attempt them.

So while she simply stopped doing many of the things she used to enjoy, there are two of the most basic day to day tasks imaginable, that she did struggle with, that really stand out in my mind.

Firstly she couldn't hang clothes on a coat hanger. She would stand with a shirt in one hand and a coat hanger in the other trying to work out the next step. She would eventually drape the shirt on the hanger and it would immediately fall off. After a couple of attempts, she would then dump the shirt and the hanger in the bottom of the wardrobe. Each day I would hang everything back up (trousers, shirts etc. together, in colour coordinated order to try and help her choose what to wear the following day) and the next day it would look like a bomb had been dropped again.

The second thing that sticks in my mind was her complete inability to make a cup of tea or coffee. She would go through some of the steps but very rarely in the right order. So for example, sometimes she would put sugar in the cup but forget the coffee or she would put the coffee in the kettle (rather than the cup) or she would put the water (sometimes warm, sometimes cold) straight into the coffee jar completely bypassing the need for cups. It really is quite amazing the number of variations there are to incorrectly make a cup of tea or coffee.

At the very beginning, we would try to tell Mum where she was going wrong or step in to help – take over if I am honest because there was a lot of coffee getting wasted! But this would cause Mum to get very embarrassed, which would manifest itself in agitation and then aggression if the situation couldn't be diverted. Whilst there is no easy solution, I eventually tried to discretely assist Mum. So for example with making a coffee, I would say, "Is the kettle full?" prompting her to check and then I would hand her the cups, therefore making sure they remained a step in the process and so on and this often helped.

I also think it helps just understanding that something as simple as making a cup of coffee will be become difficult, very quickly, for someone with dementia with Lewy bodies and that they are not doing it on purpose. In the early days, we simply didn't understand why she was struggling so much with something so simple and probably got quite frustrated as a result.

35. Lewy who: Motor problems

Up to two-thirds of people with dementia with Lewy bodies develop motor (movement) problems at some point.

The movement problems they experience are similar to those of Parkinson's disease and include slowness and rigidity of movement, problems with balance and walking is often stooped and shuffling. Symptoms can be as severe as in Parkinson's but usually milder. Tremor may also appear but is much less common and less severe than in Parkinson's.

Shortly before Mum started with the symptoms of dementia, she complained about stiff and painful joints. Rheumatoid Arthritis was diagnosed, a condition that causes pain, swelling and stiffness in the joints, usually in the hands, feet and wrists. Mum's pain did seem to be primarily in her hands but she also complained of pain in her arms and shoulders, and I now wonder whether the stiffness was related to her dementia. Having said that, a drug called Sulfasalazine used to treat Rheumatoid Arthritis was prescribed, which did seem to help.

So right from the start of her cognitive problems Mum suffered from stiff limbs, either as a result of Rheumatoid Arthritis or dementia with Lewy bodies or both.

Mum's stiffness got worse as her illness progressed and everyday tasks like dressing became more difficult. It was while living at Rivermead that Mum started to need help dressing – before she needed help choosing what to wear but once laid out she could usually manage herself with a little guidance. One day a nurse advised me that Mum had started lashing out while they were trying to dress her and so they had arranged a meeting with the Community Psychiatric Nurse for advice.

Now I knew from experience that you had to be gentle when helping Mum to dress as she obviously experienced pain if you tried to manhandle her too much. So I suggested that she was given regular pain relief before they tried to dress her and a couple of weeks later the situation was much improved.

Also from early on in her illness Mum was unsteady on her feet and her balance became more of an issue as the disease progressed. The problem was always exasperated if she was unwell.

In the later stages of dementia with Lewy bodies, a person becomes unable to turn or change direction quickly. I learnt from experience that you had to be very careful with Mum, because if you were behind her, and you called her name, she would spin around, lose her balance and almost always fall.

Falls became a more common problem and in the last few months of her life, Mum had several falls. Each time this happened the care home would call an ambulance who would advise a trip to hospital as a precaution. Now I may have mentioned that Mum hated hospitals and any visits would cause severe upset and distress. Thankfully, we managed to persuade the care home to avoid a hospital visit wherever possible. On one occasion however, she banged her head so a hospital trip was unavoidable and as expected Mum was terrified and therefore became aggressive and difficult.

Tremors were never a massive issue with Mum, however in the later stages, a noticeable tremor would occur while she was eating. Not a problem particularly but it did mean that she (and often me) would end up with more food down herself than in her mouth. One way around this was for her to use her fingers, rather than a knife and fork or spoon. Whilst this wasn't exactly the best etiquette, you really do get to the stage where you stop worrying about the small stuff, it was more important that she was getting enough to eat.

As dementia with Lewy bodies progresses the motor symptoms, similar to Parkinson's, become worse and so a person with advanced dementia with Lewy bodies will experience:

- ✓ Extreme rigidity. Very tense and stiff muscles will make movement very difficult.
- ✓ Poor coordination. This, together with movement problems, can lead to more frequent falls.
- ✓ Sensitivity to touch. People with advanced dementia with Lewy bodies may find even very gentle touch extremely uncomfortable.
- ✓ Difficulty speaking. Towards the later stages, they will have little to no verbal communication

and the speech that they may have will
be extremely quiet and highly unintelligible.

✓ Problems with swallowing, making eating and
drinking extremely difficult (see chapter 28).

36. Lewy who: Visual perception and illusions

People with dementia with Lewy bodies often visually misinterpret objects which seem to move or zoom towards/away from them or change shape. They also struggle with depth perception, directional sense and illusions may occur.

In the earlier stages of the disease, Mum was forever bumping into things, a problem which got worse as the disease progressed. If you were out for a walk with her, she would just walk in a straight line, paying absolutely no attention to what was in her path. You therefore had to walk arm in arm with her, manoeuvring her around people, pushchairs, benches, dogs and up and down kerbs.

Walking up and especially down steps was a particular problem. She would stand at the top of the stairs and you could almost see her trying to gauge how far down the step and wide the tread was. She would eventually just stick her foot out and drop, often missing and stumbling as a result. This problem got worse as the disease progressed and it came to the point where she was simply unable to manage stairs. If we occasionally and unexpectedly came across a couple of stairs, I would stand directly in front of Mum, on the first stair she would miss, and I would then 'piggyback' her down the rest. In the later stages, I would never have attempted more than three stairs with Mum on my own.

The problem with visual perception in relation to stairs

is an important point to remember when considering the living arrangements for someone with dementia with Lewy bodies. I believe it would have been very dangerous if Mum had had unsupervised access to stairs. There is almost no doubt in my mind, that in the later stages of Mum's illness, if she had attempted any stairs on her own, she would have fallen down from near the top – she may have hit the top step but wouldn't have managed the second. The fact that Mum's home (before going into care) was over three floors, was a big contributing factor in her going into a care home as early as she did.

Another problem was Mum's hand to mouth coordination. She would lift a spoon to her mouth and completely miss. She also really struggled with brushing her hair because she couldn't co-ordinate the hand holding the brush, to connect to her head.

Mum also suffered from illusions (when someone sees one thing as something else) and again from early on in her illness. When she was still at home I would often find her sat on the sofa with a cushion on her knee, stroking it and talking to it, obviously under the impression it was a cat.

Mum's problems with visual/spatial awareness and illusions, weren't helped by the fact that she needed glasses to correct her distance vision but was forever losing them. While she was living at home we would usually, eventually find them but once she went into Cross Lane it was like finding a needle in a haystack.

She was in hospital for four months and lost three pairs of glasses and after losing the fourth pair at Rivermead within a matter of months, we had to concede defeat.

Other than trying to ensure that a person with dementia is wearing the correct glasses, other ways to help are:

- ✓ Try not to make too many changes to the person's environment (e.g. keep furniture and other items in the same place). This can help the person feel confident moving around the home.
- ✓ Use signage to highlight important areas of the home like the toilet.
- ✓ Improve lighting levels which can reduce visual difficulties and help to prevent falls.
- ✓ Keep lighting levels even and bright to minimise shadows. Some people resist going near dark areas in corridors and rooms.
- ✓ Try to avoid 'busy' patterns (e.g. on the walls or floors) and changes in floor patterns or surfaces. They may be seen as an obstacle or barrier and the person may avoid walking in these areas.
- ✓ Reduce the risk of trips and falls by removing clutter and obstacles.
- ✓ Remove or replace mirrors and shiny surfaces if they cause problems. Some people can misinterpret a shiny surface as water.
- ✓ Close curtains or blinds at night.

37. Lewy who: Falls in blood pressure & dizziness

Dementia with Lewy bodies affects the nervous system, which can cause orthostatic hypotension (also known as postural hypotension). Orthostatic hypotension is a form of low blood pressure that occurs when you stand up from sitting or lying down.

Orthostatic hypotension is caused because not enough blood is reaching the brain because sensors in the carotid arteries and aorta don't respond to falling blood pressure. The heart fails to beat faster and as a result blood pools in the lower half of the body due to gravity.

Symptoms include becoming lightheaded or dizzy, vision may become grey or dark and in extreme cases, people faint. Other symptoms include weakness, fatigue, nausea, palpitations and headache.

Mum would always feel dizzy and sway on standing up. At first, we didn't appreciate it was a symptom of dementia with Lewy bodies – in fact this happened well before we got a diagnosis. If we were out, for example having lunch in a cafe or pub, her dizziness always seemed to be worse than usual when she stood up to leave (possibly because it was a warm and busy environment). As a result, Mum started having panic attacks.

Later in her illness, once I understood that it was a physical symptom of her dementia, I used to always try to help Mum up gradually, rather than her standing up too quickly. I would then always make sure she stood still for a minute or so before setting off. If she was having a particularly bad dizzy spell, I would stand in front of her, make her put her hands on my shoulders and focus on me. Making her focus seemed to help make the dizziness pass.

Orthostatic hypotension can be caused by many different conditions including dehydration. As Mum's condition progressed it became more and more difficult to get her to take enough fluids, which I can only imagine, exasperated the problem, as Mum suffered from dizziness on standing from very early on in her illness right until the end of her life.

Dizziness on standing is one factor, along with movement and visual perception problems, why people with dementia with Lewy bodies suffer from frequent falls.

I think it is easy to underestimate how frightening dizziness can be, having the sensation that you or your environment is whirling or moving about. It definitely had a dramatic effect on Mum, although I don't think I appreciated it at the time. As well as having panic attacks, I think it was a significant factor in Mum's mood, causing her to feel depressed and not in control.

The impact it had on Mum, which I only appreciate on reflection, is why I was keen to include this chapter. Feeling dizzy every time you stand up is easy to overlook in a long list of more dramatic symptoms, such as hallucinations and fluctuating cognition, but it can have a significant impact.

38. Lewy who: REM sleep behaviour disorder

Rapid eye movement (REM) sleep, is a kind of sleep that occurs at intervals during the night and features rapid eye movements, more dreaming and bodily movement, and faster pulse and breathing.

REM sleep behaviour disorder, is a sleep disorder in which you physically act out vivid, often unpleasant dreams with vocal sounds and sudden, often violent arm and leg movements during REM sleep.

In most people, the brain turns off muscle activity during our REM sleep. However, in people with REM sleep behaviour disorder, the part of the brain that 'paralyses' them is damaged, allowing them to move about.

REM sleep behaviour disorder, may be one of the first symptoms of Parkinson's disease or a Lewy body dementia. Doctors have recognized that patients may have REM sleep behaviour disorder, years before other symptoms of Parkinson's or a Lewy body dementia appear. While not everyone with REM sleep behaviour disorder will go on to develop Parkinson's disease or a Lewy body dementia, a significant proportion do.

Dr. Bradley Boeve, Mayo Clinic researcher and LBDA Scientific Advisory Council member and his colleagues examined the medical histories of a group of patients at the Mayo Clinic with REM sleep behaviour disorder who then developed neurodegenerative diseases such as Parkinson's disease or a Lewy body dementia at least

15 years later. Among this group of patients, the median interval between the two diagnoses was 25 years, and in one patient the interval was 50 years (i.e. they suffered from REM sleep behaviour disorder 15 - 25 years before they suffered from a Lewy body disease).

I have included this chapter, because for as long as I can remember, Mum has talked and moved about in her sleep i.e. decades before she became ill with dementia with Lewy bodies. It was always a bit of a joke in our family and when Mum and I used to go and visit my sister, both Kate and I would refuse to stay in the same room as Mum. It really was quite alarming when she would sit up in bed and start talking. It used to scare me to death.

Obviously back then we didn't have a label for it (i.e. REM sleep behaviour disorder), and we certainly didn't know that it was a possible precursor to dementia with Lewy bodies. So while not everyone who suffers from REM sleep behaviour disorder will go on to develop a Lewy body disease, Mum was one of the ones who did. Tragically it seems, it was already 'written in the stars.'

But the fact that the connection between REM sleep behaviour disorder as a precursor to a Lewy body disease has been made, is really positive. Because if an effective preventative measure is devised, it could be given at the first sign of REM sleep behaviour disorder.

39. Dementia: The 7 A's of dementia

The following are 7 common symptoms of dementia, known as the 7 A's for obvious reasons.

- ✓ Anosognosia (no knowledge of illness).
- ✓ Aphasia (loss of language).
- ✓ Agnosia (loss of recognition).
- ✓ Apraxia (loss of purposeful movement).
- ✓ Amnesia (loss of memory).
- ✓ Altered perception (loss of visual perception).
- ✓ Apathy (loss of initiation).

Mum suffered from all 7 symptoms but not everyone will, as it will depend on which part of the brain has been affected by disease. For example, anosognosia is caused by damage/changes to the brain's frontal lobe which is responsible for our self-image, whereas aphasia is caused by damage to the left side of the brain responsible for language.

Below is a more in-depth look at the 7 A's of dementia.

Anosognosia is the medical term given to someone with a mental illness who is unaware of their condition.

Mum was in complete denial about her illness and initially, I thought that it was because she was embarrassed about her diagnosis. Mum often used to ask, "Explain to me why you think I have dementia?" Although there is no doubt that Mum was embarrassed by her illness, I now believe that she was also genuinely unaware that she was ill.

I wish that I had known about anosognosia in the earlier stages of Mum's illness as I would have approached her questions differently, if I had realized that she had a genuine lack of insight.

Aphasia is the term used to describe someone who has difficulty with language and speech, including problems with reading, listening, speaking and writing (see chapter 23). There are 4 broad categories of aphasia:

- ✓ Expressive aphasia (non-fluent) is where someone has difficulty communicating their thoughts and ideas.
- ✓ Receptive aphasia (fluent) is where someone has difficulty understanding things.
- ✓ Anomic aphasia is where someone has difficulty finding the right names for people, objects or places.
- ✓ Global aphasia is the most severe form of aphasia where someone loses almost all language function including the ability to speak, understand speech, read or write.

Agnosia is the term given when someone is unable to process sensory information, leading to an inability to recognize objects, people, smells, shapes, or sounds even though, for example, there is no damage to a person's hearing or sight. There are 3 categories of agnosia:

- ✓ Auditory agnosia is the inability to recognize or differentiate between sounds.

- ✓ Tactile agnosia is the inability to recognize or identify objects by touch alone.
- ✓ Visual agnosia is the inability to recognize objects.

There are many types of each category of agnosia, for example:

- ✓ A type of auditory agnosia is phonagnosia, which is the inability to recognize familiar voices.
- ✓ A type of tactile agnosia is autotopagnosia, which is the inability to orient to parts of the body.
- ✓ A type of visual agnosia is prosopagnosia (also known as face blindness), which is the inability to recognize a familiar face.

Apraxia is the inability to carry out skilled movement, such as perform known tasks, even though the instruction has been understood and the person has the physical ability to do so. There are several kinds of apraxia including:

- ✓ Buccofacial or orofacial apraxia is the inability to carry out facial movements on command such as licking lips, whistling, coughing, or winking.
- ✓ Limb-kinetic apraxia is the inability to make fine, precise movements with an arm or leg.
- ✓ Ideomotor apraxia is the inability to make the proper movement in response to a verbal command.

- ✓ Ideational apraxia is the inability to make multiple, sequential movements, such as dressing, eating, and bathing.
- ✓ Verbal apraxia is difficulty coordinating mouth and speech movements.
- ✓ Constructional apraxia is the inability to copy, draw, or construct simple figures.
- ✓ Oculomotor apraxia is difficulty moving the eyes on command.

Amnesia is a condition that results in memory loss or the inability to form new memories, and memory loss is a common symptom in some types of dementia. Types of amnesia include:

- ✓ Anterograde amnesia is the inability to form new memories.
- ✓ Retrograde amnesia is where someone will lose existing, previously made memories.
- ✓ Transient global amnesia (TGA) is where someone experiences fluctuating confusion or agitation over the course of several hours. They may experience memory loss in the hours before the attack, and will probably have no lasting memory of the experience.

Altered perception is the inability to interpret sensory information. For example, someone with dementia may suffer from problems with depth perception, where they are unable to correctly judge the distance of an object to themselves, which can result in bumps and falls.

Mum had a particular problem with steps as she was unable to gauge how far down the step or wide the tread was and she would nearly always stumble.

Apathy is defined as a lack of interest, enthusiasm or concern. There are many reasons why someone with dementia will suffer from apathy including problems in the brain's motivation pathways or a decreased function (for example an inability to initiate conversation or perform certain tasks).

Mum appeared to suffer from apathy from early on in her illness but it is likely that the reason was more her inability to perform certain tasks rather than a lack of interest.

40. Our story: The 10 most important things I learnt

Caring for someone with dementia can be frustrating, stressful, heartbreaking and completely overwhelming and the following are the 10 most important things that I learnt the hard way. Although they are often easier said than done, I believe that if you don't, you will only be exasperating the behaviours that make dementia so difficult to deal with in the first place. They are all things that had I known earlier, they would have made the journey easier for all of us, but especially for Mum.

1. As soon as you are concerned that a loved one may have dementia, make sure you have a basic understating, not only about dementia in general, but about the specific diseases that cause it. This will help you work with their doctor to get an accurate diagnosis. Once the type of dementia has been diagnosed, **learn as much as you possibly can**, because once you understand the symptoms, the less confusing and overwhelming they become.

2. From very early on in her illness Mum used to hallucinate, which before we learnt that hallucinations are a common symptom of dementia with Lewy bodies, were very alarming. In the early days, we used to spend hours trying to convince her that there was nobody living in her house, which just led to upset and mistrust. I eventually learnt that **their hallucinations are very real to them** and with

Mum, the best way to deal with it was to try and distract her onto something else, usually by asking her if she wanted to go for a coffee.

3. In the early days, we tried to keep Mum engaged in the things she used to enjoy, like cooking, even though she seemed disinterested and would wander off. I now understand that because of the disease, she was unable to carry out the simplest tasks, and trying to encourage her just led to embarrassment, frustration and a loss of self-confidence. It is important that you **understand their limitations.**

4. **Never put someone with dementia in the back of a car alone, especially at night.** Once Mum, my partner and I went to see my sister and on the way back Mum sat in the back. It was a journey of a couple of hours and when we set off it was light but soon became dark. About halfway through the journey I turned to ask Mum if she was ok, to which she replied that she was terrified and needed to get out of the car. She was so terrified that we eventually had to stop the car and I got in the back with her.

5. **Do not constantly correct or try and make someone with dementia remember things**. You have to accept that if they can't remember your name, for example, it doesn't mean that they don't love you. It simply means that the part of the brain responsible for memory has been destroyed by disease. Constantly reminding them is not going to make them

remember, it is only going to embarrass and upset them.

6. **Go with the flow, do not get hung up on the little things and never be embarrassed**. In the early days, if Mum had her jumper on back to front, for example, I would spend ages trying to persuade her to change, leading to upset and agitation. As the disease progressed and just getting her dressed was a monumental effort, I stopped doing this and concentrated on the things that really mattered like was she content, eating enough and pain-free.

7. **Never ignore, talk through, over or about someone with dementia as though they are not there.** This is something that I always tried very hard not to do but I have seen others do it, time and time again, and I have seen the impact it had on Mum. Try and remember that just because someone with dementia may struggle to articulate what they think, doesn't mean that they don't have a point to make. Try and find ways to help them.

8. **Keep trying different approaches when dealing with changes in behaviour** until you find a technique that works. I always found that distraction, by asking Mum if she wanted to go for 'coffee and cake' usually worked.

9. **It is unfair to argue with someone with dementia** as they no longer have the ability to apply logic and rational thought to a situation. I always feel that arguing with them is like

arguing with a small child and is really unfair and cruel.

10. **Be careful what you say as an innocent comment can be overheard and misinterpreted** into something frightening. Once Mum accidentally overheard us updating a family member that she had been sectioned during her stay in Cross Lane hospital. This absolutely terrified her as she was convinced she was going to prison and kept asking over and over again what she had done wrong.

Finally, **remember that love will endure**. They may no longer be able to articulate how they feel, they may forget your name, but this does not mean they no longer love you. Try and help them find other ways of expressing themselves such as a cuddle or even a simple smile.

41. Lewy who: Important information

In this chapter, I wanted to share information that I feel is important for anyone with, or caring for someone with, dementia with Lewy bodies.

Why symptoms may deteriorate?
One of the key symptoms of dementia with Lewy bodies is fluctuating cognition i.e. changes in awareness and concentration where someone will swing from a state of alertness to appearing drowsy and/or confused.

However, in addition, the following will also cause the symptoms of dementia with Lewy bodies to significantly deteriorate:

- ✓ Physical illness such as a urine or chest infection.
- ✓ Stress or anxiety.
- ✓ Changes to medication – this can include changing the dosage of existing medication or introducing new dementia related medication. Even changing the time at which the medication is administered can have an impact. People with dementia with Lewy bodies are also often sensitive to prescription and over the counter medication for non dementia related conditions.

Note: Antipsychotic drugs can also have a severe impact on someone with Lewy body dementia, see chapter 16 for more details.

Whenever Mum was either physically ill, stressed or had her medication changed the impact would be:

- ✓ Significantly increased confusion.
- ✓ More powerful hallucinations.
- ✓ Extreme tiredness.
- ✓ More unsteady on feet, especially on standing up.
- ✓ Worsening hand tremors.
- ✓ Decreased coordination i.e. difficulty lifting cup to mouth.
- ✓ Weakening voice.
- ✓ Experienced greater stiffness and pain.

It is therefore important that if you are caring for someone with dementia with Lewy bodies you:

- ✓ Consult with a doctor at the first sign of illness; do not wait for the symptoms to subside.
- ✓ Try and keep stress and anxiety to a minimum. With Mum, we found that she was simply unable to do the things she previously enjoyed, such as cooking, and trying to encourage her to continue caused stress and anxiety.
- ✓ If dementia related medication (or the dosage) is being changed, plan for a decline in the dementia related symptoms.
- ✓ Try and administer medication at the same time every day.
- ✓ Consult with your doctor before introducing any over the counter medication.

Capgras syndrome

Capgras syndrome is named after Joseph Capgras (1873-1950), a French psychiatrist who first described the disorder in 1923. Capgras syndrome, also known as Capgras delusion, is the irrational belief that a familiar person or place has been replaced with an exact duplicate, an imposter.

Delusions, or false beliefs, are common in Lewy body dementias and Capgras syndrome, according to one study, affects approximately 17% of people with dementia with Lewy bodies.

Mum suffered from Capgras syndrome and was convinced that her house wasn't her own home and that we had sold her house and moved her to a new one without her consent. This was particularly challenging to deal with as no amount of reasoning could persuade her otherwise. I now realize that it was pointless trying to convince her and that we would have been better trying to distract her onto something else.

Insight

Unlike other forms of dementia, people with dementia with Lewy bodies experience fluctuations in their cognition and memory and so they have periods of lucidity right through to the end of their life.

The word 'insight' (which means the capacity to gain an accurate and deep understanding of someone or something) is a term I have heard used to describe Mum when she had moments of clarity, amid the usual confusion of her mind.

Mum used to have many periods of 'insight' when she would say the most sensible or profound statement out of nowhere. Once we were having a chat and Mum wasn't making much sense and I had a little chuckle to myself when she suddenly said, "I hope you're not been facetious?" which made me laugh even more.

I replied, "I don't think so but I'm not sure I even know what it means."

To which she replied, "It means cheeky, and you are."

Another time we were sat in the garden and we had been chatting when I said, "I know Mum, what's life all about?" Not sure what we were chatting about but it must have been profound!

Mum replied, clear as day, "Its precious is what it is and you must never forget it." Priceless!

Clinically, patients with a Lewy body dementia may have more insight into their cognitive deficits when compared to patients with Alzheimer's disease. When Mum first arrived at Rivermead, the staff told me that she would often have real insight about her dementia and she would ask questions about whether she had dementia and how they knew. Often she would get very upset but would insist on talking it through.

Once, when we were sat chatting Mum said to me, "But I am no good to you now, not like this." I remember that tears immediately sprang to my eyes, it was so heartbreaking. After I had reassured her that she was the best Mum in the world she said, "Really, well that's good then."

So while some 'insights' can be upsetting for everyone, it can also be very rewarding when you get to glimpse the person of old and are left with new cherished memories.

42. Just Be Dementia Friendly

Throughout my journey with Mum, I have been struck by key points to remember, both when helping someone with dementia to live with the respect and dignity they deserve, but also things to hang onto when times seem bleak. Quotes to remind you to 'Just Be Dementia Friendly.'

- ✓ One of the easiest ways to rob someone with dementia of their dignity is to be dismissive. To talk through, over or about them as though they are not there. Include, involve and respond as though you understand, even when you don't.
- ✓ People in the later stages of dementia need help with every aspect of their daily lives, from getting up, toileting, dressing, all aspects of personal hygiene, eating, drinking and sitting in a chair. Everything becomes a monumental, time-consuming effort. But throughout it all, we must try and ensure that they are treated with kindness, dignity and respect.
- ✓ I believe that dementia takes a person's memories. It takes their ability to communicate, perform daily tasks, takes their freedom of choice. But it can't take their values, their inherent personality. They hang on to those and so must we.
- ✓ People with advancing dementia struggle to live in our reality. They no longer understand our language or social barriers. They see and hear things differently. See things that we cannot. For

them, ours is a land of confusion. So if they can no longer live in our reality, then we must learn how to connect with them in theirs.

- ✓ When dealing with a loved one with dementia, remember the person and not the disease. When dealing with changes in behaviour, remember it's the disease and not the person.

- ✓ Some people say, "They don't even know who I am, what's the point of visiting?" I say, "How are they ever supposed to remember who you are, if you never visit."

- ✓ Following dementia, some people say, "They are not the person they were." But just because they can no longer articulate their opinions, thoughts and feelings, doesn't mean they don't have any. Help them find new ways of expressing themselves.

- ✓ Relationships do change following dementia and like any relationship, you get what you give. If you are argumentative, frustrated and dismissive, you will get agitation, upset and disengagement. If you are patient, kind and inclusive, you will get love, laughter and trust.

- ✓ Sometimes the behaviour of people with dementia can be different to the 'norm.' They may have their jumper on back to front. They may talk to themselves. They may put sugar on their chips. They may say things, others would only think. Try not to be embarrassed and educate others not to be as well.

✓ I believe the sooner you stop involving someone with dementia in the decision making processes, the more you correct them. The sooner they will lose their confidence, their sense of self. Then the sooner the symptoms such as agitation and depression will take hold.

43. Final Note

So ours was a journey of roughly 7 years. There were some very dark times, especially in the early days when Mum was at home and we didn't really understand what we were dealing with. Her time in Cross Lane was also extremely difficult as Mum was so anxious and agitated it was truly heartbreaking. The decision to put Mum in a home and finding a suitable one was also heartbreaking, but ironically she seemed to settle into the home well and to some degree we got our old Mum back. I have some lovely memories of the times I spent with her there, when we used to go for a coffee or a stroll around the local pond. Or we would simply sit and chat, incomprehensible conversations that could last for hours.

I know it sounds dramatic but I do feel traumatised by Mum's illness and subsequent death. I think about Mum every morning when I awake and every night when I close my eyes. But I have to fight to remember the happy times, when more often it's the heartbreaking ones that crowd my head. I have to force myself to remember the lovely smile and the love that never died, rather than the last few days of her life or the times when she was anxious and distressed.

Dementia is a truly awful disease that is still greatly misunderstood. It never ceased to amaze me when I told people that Mum had dementia, how many asked, "Does she know who you are?" as though memory loss is the only symptom. I was lucky because right to the end of her life, although she didn't always get my name right, she always recognized me as someone she knew and loved and I would always get a big smile and a hug. So in answer to that question I always reply, "Yes she does, in the only way that matters."

I think one of the hardest things to cope with if a loved one has dementia is just how vulnerable they become. As her disease progressed Mum became totally vulnerable, dependant on others for all aspects of daily living and unable to assess situations which were potentially dangerous. We were lucky that Mum was in a home that we had confidence in, where we knew that she wouldn't be mistreated or taken advantage of, but I know others aren't always as lucky.

Mum had always been a very strong person, but she was also very private and largely kept her feelings to herself. After she got ill, she tended to open up more, sharing things that she had kept private her whole life, things I would perhaps rather have not known. So although I have some awful memories that will haunt my dreams forever, I also have precious ones. I have memories of two Mums. The strong and confident one, who before she got ill always fought my battles. And the one who, following dementia, still showed amazing strength of character but also showed a softer and often highly amusing side. I love the memories of these two Mums in an equal, albeit different way and strangely I am thankful that I got to meet both of them.

Dementia not only affects the person with the disease

but also has a dramatic impact on the whole family. Dementia has the potential to rip families apart. We were lucky that we survived Mum's journey but we came close to crumbling a time or two. But although we survived, our family will never be the same again because the glue that held it together has gone. The light that guided our way slowly faded over seven agonising years.

More than anything I wish Mum hadn't had to endure the horrific disease that is dementia with Lewy bodies. I wish that she hadn't had her life cruelly snatched away at the relatively young age of 67. I wish she was still with us. But she did get the disease and she is no longer with us so all I can do now is try to make sure something good comes from it.

Throughout Mum's journey, I have met some amazing people. I have nothing but thanks and admiration for the doctors, nurses and carers who all dealt with Mum with kindness and respect. Before Mum got ill I had never been touched by dementia and my view was probably rather ignorant and stigmatized. However, I am now in awe of the many people I have met who are living with dementia who have changed my perception with their warmth and humour.

As a result of Mum's illness, I believe I am a better person, more compassionate, less prejudiced and more willing to help others. I am also committed to raising awareness about dementia, especially Lewy body dementia, to try and help others going through their own journey. I also believe that raising awareness is the only way to combat the stigma that is still attached to dementia, the only way to promote a dementia friendly society.

Mum was very ashamed of her dementia and I do worry that she would have resented the fact that I am sharing our journey. But she was also a kind person who would always do what she could to help others. She was also a great advocate for education, so I hope she would understand why I am sharing our story, to educate and help others improve their journey.

I know that I did the very best I could for Mum, with the information I had at the time, and that brings some comfort amid the overwhelming feeling of grief and loss. So although our journey is now at an end, for those of you who are still on your Lewy body dementia journey, I hope you have found this book interesting and useful. I would urge you again to learn as much as you can about the disease and never give up on your loved one. Remember however bleak things may seem, love really does conquer all and Mum proved that to me time and time again right up until her last breath.

Journey's End.

44. References

The following websites have provided invaluable information both to me personally throughout Mum's journey and as a source of information included in this book.

Alzheimer's Society.

https://www.alzheimers.org.uk/

- ✓ A source of information on dementia.
- ✓ A source of information on how to support someone with visual perceptual difficulties.

Alzheimer's Research UK.

http://www.alzheimersresearchuk.org/

- ✓ A source of information on dementia.
- ✓ A source of information on drugs used in dementia care.

Alzheimer's Association.

http://alz.org/

- ✓ A source of information on dementia.
- ✓ A source of information on the differences between Alzheimer's disease and dementia with Lewy bodies.
- ✓ As source of information on sundowning.

Lewy Body Dementia Association.

https://www.lbda.org/

- ✓ A source of information on Lewy body dementia.
- ✓ A source of information on antipsychotic drugs.
- ✓ A source of information on the impact of LBD on the family caregiver.
- ✓ A source of information on REM sleep behaviour disorder.
- ✓ A source of information on Capgras syndrome.

The Lewy Body Society.

http://www.lewybody.org/

- ✓ A source of information on Lewy body dementia.
- ✓ A source of information on fluctuating cognition, visual hallucination and perception.

Parkinson's UK.

https://www.parkinsons.org.uk/

- ✓ A source of information on Parkinson's disease.

Mayo Clinic.

http://www.mayoclinic.org/

- ✓ A source of information on orthostatic hypotension.
- ✓ A source of information on REM sleep behaviour disorder.

Made in United States
Orlando, FL
21 February 2022